Down's Syndro
Reproductive Poiitics

MW01167276

In the UK and beyond, Down's syndrome screening has become a universal programme in prenatal care. But why does screening persist, particularly in light of research that highlights pregnant women's ambivalent and problematic experiences with it?

Drawing on an ethnography of Down's syndrome screening in two UK clinics, Thomas explores how and why we are so invested in this practice and what effects this has on those involved. Informed by theoretical approaches that privilege the mundane and micro practices, discourses, materials, and rituals of everyday life, *Down's Syndrome Screening and Reproductive Politics* describes the banal world of the clinic and, in particular, the professionals contained within it who are responsible for delivering this programme. In so doing, it illustrates how Down's syndrome screening is 'downgraded' and subsequently stabilised as a 'routine' part of a pregnancy. Further, the book captures how this routinisation is deepened by a systematic, but subtle, framing of Down's syndrome as a negative pregnancy outcome. By unpacking the complex relationships between professionals, parents, technology, policy, and clinical practice, Thomas identifies how and why screening is successfully routinised and how it is embroiled in both new and familiar debates surrounding pregnancy, ethics, choice, diagnosis, care, disability, and parenthood.

The book will appeal to academics, students, and professionals interested in medical sociology, medical anthropology, science and technology studies (STS), bioethics, genetics, and/or disability studies.

Gareth M. Thomas is a Lecturer in Sociology in the School of Social Sciences at Cardiff University. He is a sociologist who is interested in – among other things – medicine, disability, stigma, reproduction, health and well-being, technology, place, and interaction.

Routledge Studies in the Sociology of Health and Illness

Available titles include:

Institutionalizing Assisted Reproductive Technologies
The Role of Science, Professionalism and Regulatory Control
Alexander Styhre and Rebecka Arman

Assisted Reproductive Technologies in the Global South and North
Issues, Challenges and the Future
Edited by Virginie Rozée and Sayeed Unisa

Down's Syndrome Screening and Reproductive Politics
Care, choice, and disability in the prenatal clinic
Gareth M. Thomas

Social Science of the Syringe
A Sociology of Injecting Drug Use
Nicole Vitellone

Forthcoming titles:

The Social Determinants of Male Health
John MacDonald

Fathering Children with Autism
Needs, Practices and Service Use
Carol Potter

Socio-economics of Personalized Medicine in Asia
Shirley Hsiao-Li Sun

Financing Healthcare in China
Towards universal health insurance
Sabrina Ching Yuen Luk

Self-Medication and Society
Mirages of Autonomy
Sylvie Fainzang

Down's Syndrome Screening and Reproductive Politics

Care, choice, and disability in the prenatal clinic

Gareth M. Thomas

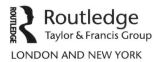
Routledge
Taylor & Francis Group

LONDON AND NEW YORK

First published 2017 by Routledge

2 Park Square, Milton Park, Abingdon, Oxfordshire OX14 4RN
52 Vanderbilt Avenue, New York, NY 10017

Routledge is an imprint of the Taylor & Francis Group, an informa business

First issued in paperback 2019

Copyright © 2017 Gareth M. Thomas

The right of Gareth M. Thomas to be identified as author of this work
has been asserted by him/her in accordance with sections 77 and 78 of
the Copyright, Designs and Patents Act 1988.

All rights reserved. No part of this book may be reprinted or
reproduced or utilised in any form or by any electronic, mechanical, or
other means, now known or hereafter invented, including photocopying
and recording, or in any information storage or retrieval system,
without permission in writing from the publishers.

Notice:
Product or corporate names may be trademarks or
registered trademarks, and are used only for identification and
explanation without intent to infringe.

British Library Cataloguing in Publication Data
A catalogue record for this book is available from the British Library

Library of Congress Cataloging in Publication Data
Names: Thomas, Gareth M., author.
Title: Down's syndrome screening and reproductive politics : care,
choice, and disability in the prenatal clinic / Gareth M. Thomas.
Other titles: Routledge studies in the sociology of health and illness.
Description: Abingdon, Oxon ; New York, NY : Routledge, 2017. |
Series: Routledge studies in the sociology of health and illness | Includes
bibliographical references and index.
Identifiers: LCCN 2016043245 | ISBN 9781138959132 (hbk) |
ISBN 9781315660806 (ebk)
Subjects: | MESH: Down Syndrome--diagnosis | Prenatal Diagnosis--
ethics | Diagnostic Tests, Routine--ethics | Politics | Health Policy
Classification: LCC RJ506.D68 | NLM WS 107 | DDC 362.196/858842--
dc23
LC record available at https://lccn.loc.gov/2016043245

ISBN: 978-1-138-95913-2 (hbk)
ISBN: 978-0-367-22412-7 (pbk)

Typeset in Garamond
by Taylor & Francis Books

To Alison and Martin, the most generous and thoughtful parents that anyone could wish for. Completing the study on which this book is based would not have been possible without your understanding, kindness, and willingness to waive a few debts.

To Ivor Thomas (Grampy) – my pensive, quick-witted, and kind-hearted grandfather; and Margaret Codd (Nana) – my caring and doting grandmother. You are gone but never forgotten.

Contents

Acknowledgements   viii
Abbreviations   x
Preface   xi
Fieldnote conventions   xvii
Details of participants   xviii
Permissions   xx

1   Introduction   1

2   A short socio-history   25

3   Hands-off work   48

4   A can of worms   77

5   The elephant in the consultation room   107

6   Expectant parents, expecting perfection   143

7   Keeping the back door ajar?   173

Index   195

Acknowledgements

My first debt is to the people who worked in or used the services of Freymarsh and Springtown. Without their cooperation and benevolence, this study would not have been possible. I am enormously grateful to the professionals who generously welcomed me into an initially daunting situation and granted me access to encounters in which privacy was the original expectation. My gratitude is unending, if anonymous, for those people who, working diligently in trying circumstances, always made time for me. A special thank you is reserved for Dr Karman, one of the most generous individuals that I have ever encountered both personally and professionally. Dr Karman's kindness, composure, and commitment to providing the best possible care was a welcome presence for me, colleagues, and people using the services of Freymarsh and Springtown.

A study of this magnitude would not have been completed were it not for the help of others. My Ph.D. supervisors, Joanna Latimer and Adam Hedgecoe, were indispensable figures who provided energy, encouragement, and wise counsel since the research developed from a two-page proposal. Their constant support and attention to detail is a gift I can never reciprocate. I have profited from engaging with many scholars who have influenced and bettered this work. For their advice and recommendations, I thank — in alphabetical order — Paul Atkinson, Patrick Brown, Angus Clarke, Sara Delamont, Rebecca Dimond, Des Fitzgerald, Arthur Frank, Nicola Gale, Faye Ginsburg, Alex Hillman, Jamie Lewis, Robyn Lotto, Deborah Lupton, Rayna Rapp, Julie Roberts, Barbara Katz Rothman, Robin Smith, and Heather Strange. The comments of Susie Scott and Anne Kerr, both during and after my Ph.D. viva, have improved this book and my research more broadly. I thank Amanda Coffey, Eva Elliott, Gabrielle Ivinson, Martin Innes, Geraldine Maddison (and everyone at the Forsythia Youth Project), Emma Renold, and Gareth Williams for their collaboration, support, and trust which certainly helped to produce this book. I am also grateful to Finn Bowring for his thoroughness, help, and reassurance, especially during my undergraduate and postgraduate years. I will always be thankful for his persistence in urging me to apply for a Ph.D. and I will forever remember his comic yet telling advice imparted when writing my undergraduate dissertation: 'you have got to stop trying to write like Shakespeare and have the confidence to use your own voice'. Such wise words have guided my approach ever since. I am also indebted to the many conference attendees and anonymous journal peer-reviewers who engaged with, and improved, my ideas.

The support of postgraduate friends during the Ph.D. will not be forgotten. Thanks to Tom Slater and Victoria Silverwood for reading my thesis and organising a mock viva without any serious complaint. For their constant backing and reminders that Ph.D. life was more than sitting in front of a computer, I thank Tim Banks, David Brewster, Ralph Buiser, Wil Chivers, Sophie Davies, Constantino Dumangane, Teresa Finlay, Rob Jones, Esther Muddiman, Hannah O'Mahoney, Olivia Pearson, and Sarah Witcombe-Hayes. The backing of my great friends outside of the academy is also hugely appreciated. For offering distractions, support, and clique jokes, I thank Mark Ambrose, Rob Browne, Dean Corbisiero, Ben Cross, Scott D'Arcy, Rich Pask, Steven Pitt, Gareth Price, John Richards, Jonathan Stock, and John Young.

The study was sponsored by Cardiff University, funded by the Economic and Social Research Council (award ES/1019251/1), and supported by Antenatal Results and Choices and the Down's Syndrome Association. I extend my gratitude to each organisation for their backing, and particularly to Julian Hallett and Penny Green. I am indebted to Lynne, Chris, Lauren, and Brittany who are responsible for my first experience with Down's syndrome. Growing up with Brittany is one of the best things that ever happened to me and I thank both her and her family for inadvertently igniting my interest in a topic in which I am now so invested.

I thank my parents Alison and Martin, sister Sian, and brother-in-law Laurence for their support and humour, even if they all gently mocked my interest in becoming, in their own words, an 'ologist'. It is difficult to find words to express how thankful I am to them for everything that they have done for me. I have been exceptionally lucky to have them, as well as other family members, around me in times of both celebration and difficulty. To Nan, Grampy, Grancha, Nana, Dave, Julie, Andy, Helen, Angela, Dave, and my many, many cousins: thanks for everything. Finally, I thank Ellie, my partner, who is so supportive of my work, understanding of my commitments, and generous with her own time. Her selflessness gave me the time to dedicate to the book when required along with the distraction away from it when I needed that too. Her meticulousness in reading and editing this monograph has been hugely helpful and her unwavering belief in me is a great source of confidence and comfort. I am very fortunate to have her by my side.

The mistakes and problems remaining in this work are mine and mine alone.

Abbreviations

CVS   Chorionic villus sampling
FAD   Freymarsh antenatal department
FMD   Freymarsh foetal medicine department
MCA   Maternity care assistant
NHS   National Health Service
NT   Nuchal translucency
SAD   Springtown antenatal department
UK   United Kingdom

Preface

This is an ethnographic story about prenatal screening for Down's syndrome in the UK. My investment in this topic stems from growing up with Brittany, a now 27-year-old female who has Down's syndrome. We spent a lot of time in each other's company during childhood; I am around one year older than Brittany, meaning that we were regularly together at various social occasions organised by family and neighbours (and even by some disability-based charity organisations). As time progressed, it was clear that Brittany and I would tread different paths. In 2006, Brittany stayed in our hometown, Tamworth, with her parents (later attending college and moving into supported living with her friends) and I left to begin an undergraduate degree in sociology at Cardiff University, followed immediately by a master's degree at the same institution.

Over these four years, I became increasingly interested in the social study of health, medicine, disability, and stigma. I carried out two studies in this period influenced not just by Brittany, but by lectures and scholarly conversations around such topics. The first study, my undergraduate dissertation, explored how stigma infiltrated, or not, the lives of parents who have a child with Down's syndrome. The second, my Master's thesis, focused on how mothers of children with the condition reacted to the prenatal or postnatal diagnosis and how they subsequently constructed their identity. After productive conversations with Finn Bowring, my Master's supervisor, I decided to continue this work by undertaking a Ph.D. in sociology, once again at Cardiff University, which started in October 2010 and finished in June 2014. This book is the product of that narrative. On a subject that is so personal for those involved, an author cannot distance him/herself. There is no *view from nowhere*, as it were, and I acknowledge that this history has certainly shaped my claims within this book.

Data in the book are drawn from a Ph.D. study taking place in two UK settings: (1) Freymarsh, a large NHS teaching hospital in a metropolitan area; and (2) Springtown, a privately funded fertility clinic in an affluent area. I initially planned to conduct research only in Freymarsh (I explain my access to Springtown later), which was selected for two reasons. First, Freymarsh is a large and popular hospital with a wide variety of services used by many people from different backgrounds. Second, and most importantly, Down's syndrome screening is offered to parents-to-be at this hospital. Although a more complete account of my ethnographic story is available elsewhere (see: Thomas 2014), I offer a condensed version here. In order to secure access to Freymarsh, I had to undertake NHS ethical approval. Prior to applying for this, I decided to organise meetings with my supervisors as well as healthcare professionals, policymakers, and charity organisations to discuss the research. At various points, my vague and ambitious plans led to advice being tendered, naive objectives being quashed, and recommendations being either accepted or politely rejected. After this, I was put in contact with two people at Freymarsh: Carol (manager of the antenatal department) and Dr Karman (consultant in the foetal medicine department). After many fruitful conversations with Carol and Dr Karman, I spent six months meeting other healthcare professionals to seek support and solicit guidance on the research which became vital to fleshing out the finer details of my ethical approval application (indeed, securing access to an NHS setting begins well before navigating the treacherous waters of the application process). Nonetheless, the formal support of Carol and Dr Karman – as my gatekeepers, that is, as architects of trust and linchpins of a cohort – undoubtedly lessened the chance of the NHS ethics application being rejected. Sure enough, ethical approval for the study was granted, after some minor revisions, in November 2011.

Fieldwork began almost immediately after receiving formal permission. I entered the field with some flexible research interests, intended as a guideline rather than fixed stipulations, to guide initial observations. Ethnographers frequently enter the field as if it is *pre*-constructed, as already 'existing'. This risks making a Procrustean bed for data, imposing an unwarranted order drawn from an analyst's own interpretations about wider structures and context. As such, on walking into the doors of Freymarsh, I rejected the notion that Down's syndrome screening is something which is self-evident and, instead, embraced it as a practice fragmented across different spaces. In this 'multi-sited ethnography' (Marcus 1995: 95), I 'tracked' Down's syndrome screening inside and outside the clinic walls. In so doing, I was able to map its trajectory, reflecting how bodies in modern medical practice are fragmented and transformed into different representations across various sites.

During fieldwork, then, I entered consultation rooms, offices, hospital meetings, seminars, public symposiums, laboratories, and several sites where Down's syndrome screening is 'done'. However, the vast majority of my fieldwork was spent observing three places: Freymarsh antenatal department (FAD), Freymarsh foetal medicine department (FMD), and Springtown antenatal department (SAD). This notion of 'tracking' is important for explaining my access to Springtown (the second research site). After attending FAD and FMD for one week, Dr Karman invited me to attend a privately funded fertility clinic (Springtown) which also offered screening for Down's syndrome. Dr Karman runs the Antenatal Department at Springtown and believed that I would benefit from doing research there. Thus, Springtown was constructed by Dr Karman, not me, as a key site of interest.

I spent roughly one year collecting field data. Many hours of observations are supplemented with document analysis (e.g. policy documentation, prenatal leaflets) and sixteen interviews with healthcare professionals from FAD, FMD, and SAD. Guided by the principles of interactionism and ethnomethodology (more on theory later), I chose observations as my main method for collecting data since I was guided by an interest in producing an in-depth description of a research site and the working lives of the people within it. Whilst I gratefully draw upon the information provided by parents and others, the book explores the banal real world of the contemporary hospital, its professionals, and their daily work – and how Down's syndrome screening, specifically, is done at the everyday level. Influenced by Goffman's (1959) work on how spaces are arranged socially into front and back regions, the book opens up both the clinic's public 'frontstage' (e.g. medical consultations, waiting rooms) and private 'backstage' (e.g. offices, professional-to-professional interactions, small talk), as professionals experience and understand it, with respect to prenatal screening for Down's syndrome. Observing the frontstage alone – 'where the action is' (Goffman 1967) – is a grave error as it mistakes a part for the whole (Bosk 1992). By observing frontstage *and* backstage interactions, I reveal how the frontstage of a consultation is only one component of Down's syndrome screening and is not, on its own, a microcosm of all aspects of medical work.

Throughout the research, I was invited by professionals to escort them around the clinic and into consultations. The majority of my field data, as such, is taken from observations of consultations between professionals and parents-to-be dedicated to Down's syndrome screening. These consultations took place in both FAD, the NHS clinic, and SAD, the privately funded clinic. As such, FMD (NHS foetal medicine department) and other medical worlds (e.g. laboratories) were observed less frequently. I observed 150 consultations (75 per setting) in which screening for Down's syndrome was discussed and/or carried out. Whilst the vast majority of my arguments in this book stem from such encounters, I spent much of my time in Freymarsh and Springtown hanging out, that is, immersing myself in the culture of each setting on an informal level. I was often an active participant in various scenes, yet refraining from asking outright questions and remaining somewhat muted produced details which I would not have thought to ask myself. Thus, I observed and retained information which others in the settings often deemed trivial or taken-for-granted.

Together with exploring the everyday practices and interactions of professionals with respect to screening for Down's syndrome, I wanted to explore professionals' actions not as individuals but, rather, as situated social and cultural beings enacted and positioned by routine and institutional discourses. In short, rather than assessing professionals as failing to live up to preconceived set ideals posited by models and theories of best practice, I attended to what professionals' conduct is accomplishing, why they are accomplishing these matters over others (and how professionals might be restricted in various ways), and what socio-cultural effects they are embedded within. More specifically, I became interested in who or what is privileged and/or excluded, who is made accountable, what is figured as good or bad medical practice, the extent of 'slippage' between *informal* ways of working and *formal* accounts, how identity-work is accomplished, and what/how classifications are reproduced in everyday practices.

I made fieldnotes during consultations using either a notepad or a mobile (cellular) phone. In the office or other less organised encounters, I relied on memory and created fieldnotes as accurately as possible in the setting or imme-diately after leaving the field. Writing fieldnotes meant that, on occasions, I temporarily withdrew from the action moments after it occurred. Although observational work is sacrificed here, it is more beneficial to have fewer well-recorded and illuminating observations rather than more half-reported and less developed ones. I also opted not to use a tape recorder. I felt that its possibly invasive presence could derail the natural sequence of talk and the rhythms of social life, with professionals reluctant to reveal information otherwise shared. This could have led, in turn, to securing 'an accurate representation of a misrepresentation' (Desmond 2007: 292). As such, the majority of quota-tions presented in this book rely on my own memory and fieldnotes taken whenever appropriate and possible. These are also polished editions of messier collections. The fillers, incomplete thoughts, and pauses common in the speech of professionals and parents-to-be are deleted to recover the articulate character it fulfilled in its original oral performance.

Fieldwork, for the most part, went off without a major hitch. Professionals were overwhelmingly unobtrusive and engaging on both a professional and personal level, granting me unbridled access to their working worlds. I offer four possible reasons for this. First, my study was championed by Dr Karman and Carol. They rarely, if ever, had to explicitly vouch for my presence around the respective institution, yet my affiliated status was enough to limit questions regarding my presence and give me the authority to be there. Second, I made active efforts to keep out of the way, fill downtime with interesting conversation and engage in chitchat/jokes, and be helpful (e.g. fetching drinks, switching off the lights prior to an ultrasound scan, disposing of waste). Such efforts helped maintain relationships and gain trust; being able to offer something, however mundane, is valuable currency when seeking observational rights. Third, my age (I was 22 years old at the start of the study) and student status may have helped create an impression of naivety and of being non-threatening, possibly easing professionals' initial concerns about the presence of an 'out-sider'. Equally, I may have been mistaken for a medical student, which may have facilitated my access to carry out this study. Finally, this 'outsider' status meant that I commonly became a sounding board where professionals aired their grievances and discontents possibly withheld from colleagues and intimate others. It seems, in turn, that all of this contributed to my approval in the field. However, it is best to be humble about this since one never really knows how participants view the researcher.

Despite fieldwork progressing without major concern, there were many challenges. The research required great flexibility, patience, and a serious investment of time and energy – and, at times, it could be emotionally draining. Another particular problem of my fieldwork, and of ethnography more generally, is that I assumed those who did not wish to be observed found ways to avoid this. Professionals could merely have exercised politeness yet silently objected to my presence. Similarly, if professionals were wary of my presence and desisted from behaving *naturally*, I might wonder how much was staged for my benefit. Whilst I believe our relationship was strong enough to withstand this possibility, its manifestation cannot be completely discounted. Another issue is anonymity. I provide pseudonyms for participants and locations alongside an omission of minor details, and changing some key attributes of participants, with a view to concealing identifiable information. Yet despite pseudonyms transforming the specific into the general, those close to the scene may unmask these light cloaks. Whilst social life provides wiggle room for evading previous claims, permanent texts do not.

Another challenge concerns publishing this book. Throughout my stay at Freymarsh and Springtown, I became hugely fond of the people working there. Our interactions were never limited to what you might call professional talk; we discussed television programmes, food, love lives, family, books, local and celebrity gossip, and so on. Yet the claims of this book may occasionally reflect unfavourably on them; 'under an ethnographic microscope everyone has warts and anyone can be made to look like a monster' (Bourgois 1995: 18). My intention is not to snatch secrets and put them in the public domain. Healthcare institutions are dense settings too complex to be normatively assessed and depicted as a tale of heroes and villains or saints and sinners. My policy, then, is to provide a sympathetic but clear analytical account as opposed to passing judgement on settings, people, or situations. I intend my ethnographic account, in viewing the social life of Freymarsh and Springtown unsentimentally and without any obvious bias, to be – at the very least – a fair and accurate portrayal.

For the remainder of the book, I present a front line account that outlines my attempt to uncover the mundane patterns of professionals' working lives and how they go about their everyday business of 'doing' Down's syndrome screening. Interested in everyday working practices and general types rather than specific people, I reveal how screening for Down's syndrome occupies a key position in the politics of reproduction and explore why both scientific and medical communities are so invested in this practice. In so doing, I elucidate the interactive dance between professionals and parents-to-be together with the fundamental drama of these encounters. The ethnographic method is, at its core, good storytelling. I believe that this book, an impressionistic sketch laced with my own interpretations, contains a tale worth sharing.

Bibliography

Bosk, C.L. 1992. *All God's Mistakes: Genetic Counseling in a Pediatric Hospital*. Chicago: University of Chicago Press.

Bourgois, P. 1995. *In Search of Respect: Selling Crack in El Barrio*. Cambridge: Cambridge University Press.

Desmond, M. 2007. *On the Fireline: Living and Dying with Wildland Firefighters (Fieldwork Encounters and Discoveries)*. Chicago: University of Chicago Press.

Goffman, E. 1959. *The Presentation of Self in Everyday Life*. London: Allen Lane.

Goffman, E. 1967. *Interaction Ritual: Essays on Face-to-Face Behaviour*. New York: Doubleday.

Marcus, G.E. 1995. Ethnography in/of the world system: the emergence of multi-sited ethnography. *Annual Review of Anthropology* 24, pp. 95–117.

Thomas, G.M. 2014. *The Everyday Work of Healthcare Professionals: An Ethnography of Screening for Down's Syndrome in UK Antenatal Care*. Unpublished Ph.D. Thesis, Cardiff University.

Fieldnote conventions

[…] Words or sentences omitted
'Words used by participants'
Data have been edited to preserve anonymity.
All names of people and places are pseudonyms.

Details of participants

Table 0.1 Professionals in Freymarsh antenatal department (FAD), Freymarsh foetal medicine department (FMD), and/or Springtown antenatal department (SAD).

Name	FAD role	FMD role	SAD role
Amy	Midwife	–	–
Angela	Midwife	–	–
Annie	–	Sonographer	–
Bethan	–	–	Administrative staff
Camilla	Midwife	–	–
Dr Cassidy	–	Consultant	–
Dominique	–	–	Administrative staff
Elena	–	Head midwife	–
Emma	Midwife	Midwife	–
Esther	–	–	Sonographer
Eve	Midwife	–	–
Dr Finely	–	–	Consultant*
Fiona	–	Administrative staff	–
Francine	–	Head midwife	Nurse
Gail	Midwife	–	–
Hannah	–	–	Administrative staff
Heather	–	–	Sonographer*
Isobel	–	–	Nurse
Jennifer	MCA	–	–
Joanna	–	Head midwife	–
Jodi	–	Cardiac physiologist	–
Juliana	–	–	Administrative staff
Dr Karman	–	Consultant	Consultant

Table 0.1 (continued)

Name	FAD role	FMD role	SAD role
Keri	–	–	Nurse
Lindsay	Midwife	–	–
Lisa	Radiographer*	–	Sonographer
Lois	Midwife	Midwife	–
Maggie	Midwife	–	–
Marianne	Midwife	–	–
Martha	Midwife	–	–
Michelle	MCA	–	–
Nancy	Midwife	Midwife	–
Nicola	Midwife	–	–
Olivia	Radiographer*	–	Sonographer
Pauline	Administrative staff	–	–
Rita	Midwife	–	–
Robyn	–	Midwife	–
Rosie	MCA	–	–
Roxanne	–	Sonographer	–
Sophie	Radiographer*	–	Sonographer
Susan	Midwife	–	–
Tara	Midwife	–	–
Terri	Midwife	–	–
Toni	Midwife	–	–
Dr Torres	–	Cardiologist	–
Victoria	–	–	Nurse
Whitney	Administrative staff	–	–
Yvonne	Administrative staff	–	–

Note: * This professional had no major involvement in Down's syndrome screening in the respective institution.

Permissions

Permissions have been granted from both publishers and co-authors for the reuse of some material from the following outputs:

Latimer, J.E. and Thomas, G.M. 2015. In/exclusion in the clinic: Down's syndrome, dysmorphology, and the ethics of everyday medical work. *Sociology* 49(5), pp. 937–954.
Thomas, G.M. 2014. Prenatal screening for Down's syndrome: parent and healthcare practitioner experiences. *Sociology Compass* 8(6), pp. 837–850.
Thomas, G.M. 2015. Picture perfect: '4D' ultrasound and the commoditisation of the private prenatal clinic. *Journal of Consumer Culture* [Online first].
Thomas, G.M. 2016. An elephant in the consultation room? Configuring Down's syndrome in UK antenatal care. *Medical Anthropology Quarterly* 30(2), pp. 238–258.

Chapter 1

Introduction

It is over 150 years since John Langdon Down, an English physician, first described a group of people with a condition now known as Down's syndrome (or Trisomy 21). Down's syndrome is one of the most common chromosomal conditions in the world, affecting approximately one to two of every 1,000 live births in England and Wales alone. People with Down's syndrome are likely to have a range of symptoms including learning difficulties, shortened limbs, reduced muscle tone, restricted physical growth, a flat facial profile, and a large protruding tongue, though symptoms and prognosis vary in each case. Indeed, Down's syndrome does not 'cut all children to one mould', with the relationship between genotype and phenotype being 'lacy and intricate' (Bérubé 1996: 20–21). Whilst a common feature of Down's syndrome is the variability and inconsistency of its manifestation, the condition is often clinically defined as 'compatible with life',[1] meaning that individuals are likely to survive childbirth and can survive beyond sixty years of age (CARIS 2012).

Down's syndrome currently occupies a central position in reproductive politics, particularly in the global North. Prenatal screening for the condition is now a universal programme which has come into 'routine use, becoming embedded in, we might say, a social matrix' (Cowan 1994: 36). Whilst predicted advances of genetic screening generally may be more modest than initially expected, the range of available screening techniques for Down's syndrome and other conditions, such as Edward's syndrome (or Trisomy 18) and Patau syndrome (or Trisomy 13),[2] has steadily expanded in the UK, with parents-to-be[3] increasingly making use of techniques to assemble knowledge about the health status of a foetus/baby.[4] According to the most recent statistics, roughly 74% (N=542,312) of all parents-to-be accessing NHS services in England and Wales in 2011 opted to be screened for Down's syndrome (NHS FASP 2012), although statistics vary significantly between countries (Vassy et al. 2014).[5]

The uptake in prenatal screening has increased annually in England and Wales since 2007 (53%). Whilst 2008 and 2009 saw uptake rates of 57% and 62% respectively, an uptake rate of 70% was recorded in 2010 (NHS FASP 2012). This differs from other countries, such as the Netherlands, where uptake rates vary from 38% to 86% (van den Berg et al. 2005a) and Japan where less than 2% of all pregnant women were screened (Nishiyama et al. 2013).[6] The increase in UK uptake rates may be attributable to the recent increase in maternal age (an increase in maternal age is the only known attribute increasing the chance of a foetus being diagnosed with Down's syndrome), the risk of miscarriage decreasing on account of increasingly proficient screening technologies, and service supply factors since all mothers-to-be (rather than just mothers-to-be aged thirty-five and above, as in earlier years) are now offered screening for the condition (NHS FASP 2012; ONS 2011). In addition, a report conducted by the National Down's Syndrome Cytogenetic Register (NDSCR) claims that in 2013 in England and Wales, of the 1,232 prenatal diagnoses of Down's syndrome, 90% were terminated (N=925), 8% were live births (N=82), and 2% were natural miscarriages or stillbirths (N=20); the outcome of 205 prenatal diagnoses is unknown (Morris and Springett 2014). The proportion of terminations following a diagnosis of the condition in England and Wales has remained steady for over twenty years. From the first report in 1989 until 2013, the annual rates for termination in England and Wales have ranged from 89% to 95% (the mean rate is 92%). Buckley and Buckley (2008) claim, however, that there has been an increase of 25% over fifteen years of babies with Down's syndrome being born, suggesting that this is because parents-to-be are having children later in life when the chance of having a baby with Down's syndrome increases.

Thus, despite the heavy investment in screening and diagnosis,[7] the birth rate has not fallen but what *has* been avoided is an increase in the number of babies with the condition which may have otherwise resulted (Shakespeare 2011), with around nine out of ten prenatal diagnoses of Down's syndrome ending in a pregnancy termination. This corresponds to the work of Boyd et al. (2008) who claim that ten out of eighteen European countries have an average termination rate of 88% after a prenatal diagnosis of Down's syndrome. Similarly, in areas of Australia and select US states, the termination rates following a diagnosis are reported as 95% (Collins et al. 2008) and 74% (Natoli et al. 2012) respectively. However, it is crucial to remember that many countries do not track termination rates for Down's syndrome on a national scale, with this likely being related to local variations in laws (e.g. if a termination of pregnancy for 'foetal abnormality' is legally possible).

Previous research

When considering these statistics, it is clear just how centrally Down's syndrome screening is located in reproductive (bio)politics in the UK and beyond. My book is dedicated to unpacking this practice by drawing on an ethnographic study of Down's syndrome screening in two UK prenatal clinics. Whilst studies have examined the social significance of *diagnostic* testing for Down's syndrome (Browner and Preloran 1999; Bryant et al. 2006; Crang-Svalenius et al.

1998; Markens et al. 2010; Rapp 2000) or used the terms screening and diagnostic testing interchangeably (Green and Statham 1996; Jaques et al. 2004; Kaiser et al. 2004; Marteau 1995; Press and Browner 1997), I focus exclusively on screening for the condition, arguing that this merits critical attention in its own right. This topic has previously been the subject of academic consideration. Such work derives from many different countries (and so diverse social, cultural, economic, political, and medical contexts), uses both qualitative and quantitative methods (rarely together), focuses on screening at different periods of gestation, and stems from scholarly roots such as sociology, public health, medicine (midwifery, nursing, genetics), anthropology, psychology, and bioethics. However, most studies can be categorised as examining two core interrelated aspects of Down's syndrome screening.

First, a proliferation of studies explore decision-making process of parents-to-be and why they do or do not participate in screening.[8] Whilst many of these accounts understand consenting to Down's syndrome screening as a result of rational decision-making processes, others show how screening can be an instance of conformity rather than an expression of choice (Chiang et al. 2006; Gottfreðsdóttir et al. 2009; Markens et al. 1999; Marteau 1995; Pilnick 2004; Pilnick et al. 2004; Press and Browner 1997; Santalahti et al. 1998; Sooben 2010; Williams et al. 2005). This corresponds to parents-to-be interpreting screening as a recommended part of pregnancy surveillance (Hunt et al. 2005; Vassy 2006), how they view professionals' offer of screening as endorsing its acceptance (Heyman et al. 2006; McNeill et al. 2009; Remennick 2006), and how ultrasound scans can be viewed, first and foremost, as offering a chance for meeting the baby and for making a pregnancy seem more real rather than for prenatally detecting genetic conditions (Draper 2002; Gammeltoft and Nguyén 2007; Heyman et al. 2006; Lupton 2013; Mitchell and Georges 1998; Reed 2012). In a similar vein, Tsouroufli (2011) claims that parents-to-be opt for screening as a routine aspect of prenatal care because of their prompt processing in the hospital, because professionals endorse it as a safe test (no chance of miscarriage), and because professionals expect that they will opt for the procedure.

For Baillie et al. (2000), the naturalisation of Down's syndrome screening as a 'normal' part of pregnancy means that parents-to-be are not always aware of, or prepared for, the complex information and heavy choices associated with a screening result. Many studies, indeed, report how screening prompts feelings of fear and anxiety among parents-to-be before, during, and/or after receiving a result (Aune and Möller 2012; Green and Statham 1996; Ivry 2006; Markens et al. 1999; Marteau 1995; Pilnick et al. 2004; Remennick 2006). Strategies of managing and negotiating results include developing interpretations via metaphors (Burton-Jeangros et al. 2013) or remaining emotionally detached from a foetus in the event of decisions needing to be made around a termination of pregnancy (Remennick 2006; Williams et al. 2005). This literature demonstrates, in short, that whilst parents-to-be perhaps engage with screening to abate anxiety and receive reassurance, it can also have the opposite effect.

Second, a cluster of studies on Down's syndrome screening report on the interactions between parents-to-be and professionals, particularly concerning discrepancies of knowledge directed at the level of the intertwining rhetoric of 'informed choice' and 'non-directive care'. These concepts translate to professionals tendering medically-accurate information to parents-to-be detached from personal biases. In this context, reproductive technologies are heralded as a route to liberation since they offer parents-to-be information about, and control over, their offspring (García et al. 2008; Seavilleklein 2009). However, others show that this is not always empowering (Lippman 1994; Pilnick 2008; Rapp 2000; Rothman 1986; Williams et al. 2002c). Several studies claim that parents-to-be do not perceive their care as non-directive since the provision of information is interpreted as an explicit instruction (Browner et al. 1996; Hunt et al. 2005; Lippman 1991; Williams et al. 2002c) or as coercive and directive as opposed to being passive and facilitating (Marteau et al. 1993; Tsouroufli 2011).

Others explore how professionals encounter difficulty in remaining non-directive and ensuring informed choice when communicating information on Down's syndrome screening (García et al. 2008; Heyman et al. 2006; Pilnick et al. 2004). This stems from needing to balance both professional and private values (Anderson 1999; Farsides et al. 2004; Williams et al. 2002a), the conflict between the time professionals *have* to explain screening and the time they *need* to discuss the procedure (Sooben 2010; Vassy 2006; Williams et al. 2002a), the trouble of conveying information and the practical/ethical aspects of screening (Burton-Jeangros et al. 2013; Ekelin and Crang-Svalenius 2004; Heyman et al. 2006), communication breakdowns when the first language of parents-to-be is not the native language (Hey and Hurst 2003), and the different definitions between parents-to-be and professionals of what constitutes a 'normal result' and/or a 'normal child' (Hunt et al. 2005; Williams 2006). In addition, research identifies how professionals sometimes do not know how to best support parents-to-be (Getz and Kirkengen 2003; Williams et al. 2002a), how some parents-to-be are not aware of the key features of Down's syndrome prior to screening and testing (Williams et al. 2002e), and how they may not fully understand or have realistic expectations of screening (Burton-Jeangros et al. 2013; Gammons et al. 2010; van den Berg et al. 2005b).

This important literature identifies how the development and diffusion of prenatal screening techniques has triggered critical debates around the seemingly contradictory aspects of offering reproductive choice to – and prompting social, legal, and ethical dilemmas for – parents-to-be. This means that parents-to-be, in receipt of vital information about a pregnancy, must make serious life decisions frequently on the basis of partial knowledge (Franklin and Roberts 2006; Rapp 2000; Rothman 1986). The substance and contribution of such studies is irrefutable, yet existing insights can be subjected to a number of criticisms. First, several important voices are missing or, at least, muted. As well as studies neglecting the experiences of fathers and older mothers (i.e. those clinically defined as being of 'advanced maternal age'), the research that is chiefly focused on healthcare professionals with respect to Down's syndrome screening generates a relatively undersized literature (for exceptions, see: Ekelin and Crang-Svalenius 2004; Farsides et al. 2004; McCourt 2006; Samwill 2002; Ternby et al. 2015; Williams et al. 2002a; 2002b; 2002c; 2002d; 2002e). Second, studies are mostly based on retrospective accounts of parents-to-be and professionals. They do not, as such, explore the mundane aspects of, and meaning-making practices in, medical encounters with respect to Down's syndrome screening. By de-contextualising context-specific situations and relying on romantic conceptions of a rational experiencing individual, such work is rarely grounded in ethnographic data that captures how screening is enacted, managed, and negotiated by both professionals and parents-to-be in everyday routines (for exceptions, see: Ivry 2006; 2009; Pilnick 2004; 2008; Pilnick and Zayts 2012; Schwennesen and Koch 2012).

Third, research on Down's syndrome screening seldom discusses the condition and, in so doing, subscribes to medical definitions of Down's syndrome and disability. Sooben (2010) identifies how professionals describe Down's syndrome during consultations and Bryant et al. (2006) similarly argue that prenatal settings currently provide little opportunity for people to discuss and explore their beliefs about disability. Yet too little research has involved exploring how Down's syndrome, and disability more generally, are discussed within screening consultations and how accusations that screening fosters a belief that Down's syndrome should be prevented (Alderson 2001; Vassy 2006) play out in the clinic. This critique extends to analyses of reproductive practices and how values around disability are enacted in medicine (Latimer 2007; Rapp 2000; Shakespeare 2006) and, in turn, how scientific and medical advances promote a clear definition of which people should and should not live (Lippman 1994; Parens and Asch 2000; Rothman 1998; Wasserman and Asch 2006). Many accounts, however, frame disability as a universal category.[9] Davis (1995: xv) argues that the totalising tag of disability is an extraordinarily unstable category that denies bodily variation; 'the category "disability" begins to break down when one scrutinises who make up the disabled'. Research on prenatal screening for Down's syndrome, in turn, mostly operates within a model that obscures the complexity of different and distinctive conditions (such as Down's syndrome). What is missing, then, is critical research which unpacks these universal terms that create rigid categories of existence.

The book

This book – drawing on an ethnographic study of screening for Down's syndrome in two prenatal clinics (Freymarsh and Springtown) – bridges many of the gaps outlined above. In this account, I attend to the everyday practices and relations of professionals working in prenatal medicine and explore how Down's syndrome screening is 'done' (Garfinkel 1967) in the clinic, a site in which social, cultural, and political effects are accomplished. Taking the micro and mundane seriously, since it is through these that meanings are circulated, I show how a close ethnographic reading of everyday life in clinical settings unmasks the ongoing, complex, and different ways in which knowledge, meanings, and positions are reproduced in medical encounters. In addition, considering the context of screening,[10] I show how Down's syndrome is embroiled in the broader trend of surveillance medicine together with debates around pregnancy, ethics, family, parenthood, diagnosis, care, and disability. By unpacking the complex relationships between professionals, parents-to-be, technology, policy, and clinical practice, the book captures how the successful routinisation of a biomedical technology occurs and how this reconstitutes certain ideas and values. In short, it explores how (and why) we are so invested in screening for Down's syndrome, how it persists as a widespread medical programme, and the consequences of this for parents-to-be and the professionals offering this service.

Theoretical foundations

Before delving deep into the worlds of Freymarsh and Springtown, I outline the theoretical foundations on which the book is grounded. Whilst the study can loosely be defined as a cultural and interpretive analysis, my arguments draw upon concepts borrowed from other paradigms, meaning that my theoretical allegiance is partial and indefinite. Undoubtedly, I am influenced by ethnomethodological concerns, that is, the study of peoples' methods for producing recognisable and reasonable social orders. However, in the book, I combine ethnomethodological sensibilities with ideas and concepts from several perspectives to engage with a particular way of analysing the social life of two prenatal clinics. It is worth stressing, then, that I do not wholly buy into the worldview of one tradition. Here, I procure tools offered by different theoretical foundations to make sense of Down's syndrome screening, reflecting how the complexity of this practice cannot be handled by a single discipline or framework. Restricting analysis to one perspective would not do justice to the multiple, mundane, and messy character of everyday life in the clinic which does not always cleave at neat points. This section, thus, is my attempt to condense the disorderliness into a coherent account with reference to a collection of theoretical tropes. In so doing, I identify my position for making arguments throughout the remainder of the book.

Although I synthesise several concepts and ideas, my main aim is to analyse the mundane, familiar, and taken-for-granted 'micro' practices, routines, rhythms, and rituals of everyday clinical life which reproduce order and values. By theorising the mundane, I will show how the micro and banal help us understand the wider processes and complexities of the clinic. Rather than simply interviewing professionals about work practices, I observe the interactions between them and parents-to-be, colleagues, and others. As such, a key feature of this research involves attending to the micro-study of interaction. Erving Goffman's work is valuable here. His 'dramaturgical' (Goffman 1959) insights are united by a recurring concern with the quirks of human conduct and the strategic ways that people behave in situations. During such collective recitals, people manage impressions, maintain performances, and negotiate identities to uphold normal appearances. Such co-presence, for Goffman, corresponds to the regulation of a public order. In sum, Goffman suggests that one cannot dismiss the minute as trivial, highlighting how the intricate politics of small rules and transgressions add up to ordinary yet very powerful (and symbolic) rituals and ceremonies in everyday life.

In the context of this study, I show the extraordinariness of ordinariness, analysing the subtle scaffolding of human interaction, the character of institutions, and, more generally, how professionals make sense of their world (Goffman 1959; 1983). I examine how professionals, as 'members' (Garfinkel 1967), produce a local order as well as make shared sense of their circumstances. By treating 'practical activities, practical circumstances, and practical sociological reasoning as topics of empirical study', I capture the nuance of ordinary (and often hidden) knowledge and the 'most commonplace activities of daily life' in the clinic (Garfinkel 1967: 1). As such, I identify the role that 'background expectancies' play in constructing and controlling a local (moral) order, as a socially managed production, and in accomplishing ordinary routines in the two research sites: Freymarsh and Springtown (1967: 35). Indeed, professionals 'encounter and know the moral order as perceivedly normal courses of action-familiar scenes of everyday affairs' (1967: 35). I explore, thus, how professionals transform the taken-for-granted into the 'natural' and 'moral' facts of clinical life (1967: 35). This involves treating the obvious as a phenomenon ('topic') as opposed to an 'unexplicated resource' by examining how people 'assemble particular scenes so as to provide for one another evidence of a social order as-ordinarily-conceived' (Zimmerman and Pollner 1970: 81–83). In so doing, I recognise the value of analysing the taken-for-granted and for embracing multiplicity rather than attributing social life – contextual, historical, local, and specific – to universal laws. By analysing how meanings, orders, and routines are reproduced in two clinical settings, I identify how expectations and values at the micro-level are consolidated into wider normative codes of conduct which appear as 'natural' and 'real' (Scott et al. 2013).

Important here, too, is the concept of identity (Goffman 1959) and how professionals, primarily though their interactions with parents-to-be, engage in identity-work. The social audience is important for identity construction since the self and any adjustments thereof is not a property of the individual but arises through interactions with others. Within such situated occasions, identity is relational, amorphous, and routinely created in the reflexive actions of others. People share a world with others in which there is an ongoing correspondence between each person's meanings and interpretations (Goffman 1959). As such, I explore how professionals manage, perform, and direct interaction, that is, how they take account of others and reaffirm their identity in relation to the conventions of the clinic. Related to professionals' identity-work is their 'accounting' practices (Garfinkel 1967), namely, the ways in which people signify, describe, or explain the properties of conduct in a social situation to make what they do and who they are appear grounded, reason-able, and rational to others. People work to maintain consistency, order, and meaning in their lives, that is, to accomplish identity and membership within given groups. It is principally via language, as 'situated practices of looking-and-telling', that this is accomplished and members subsequently create a sense of reality (1967: 1). This is vital for this study as I examine how professionals account for the conduct of themselves, their colleagues, and parents-to-be – that is, how they describe interactions with parents-to-be, validate their actions, and use this to (re)construct their identity.

Another aim is to identify how the micro-physics of power are enacted in Freymarsh and Springtown. The arguments of Michel Foucault are valuable here. Foucault argues that power is not concentrated in one space or possessed by one person but, rather, is localised and fragmented, with people becoming conduits through which power is exercised. Invisible yet potent in its effects, power is realised in its reach 'into the very grain of processes and everyday life' (Foucault 1980: 39). As a productive network, power is a practical accomplishment which 'produces and traverses things, it induces pleasure, forms of knowledge, produces discourses' (1980: 119). Agreeing with Foucault that power is not just repressive but productive, not just coercive but legit-imate, I explore how power works in Freymarsh and Springtown by examining how it facilitates, mobilises, and elicits the actions of those subjected to it. This focus on disciplinary power – working consciousness through, and control-ling the operations and positions of, the body (Foucault 1973) – allows me to analyse how professionals formulate, disperse, and use power and knowledge in and across settings to organise activities and assign meanings to the conduct of themselves and others.

In this book, I capture how power is expressed and meanings are distributed in the clinic via 'discourse' (Foucault 1972), that is, in the language and practices of embodied individuals. In the prenatal clinic, discourse constructs knowledge and disciplines via the production of categories and assemblages of text, particularly around – putting it simply – the 'normal' and 'abnormal' body. People are constituted via 'dividing practices' (Foucault 1983: 208) which, as forces of 'normalising judgement' (Foucault 1973: 177), produce classifications. People can be divided, for instance, into 'the mad and the sane, the sick and the healthy, the criminals and the "good boys"' (Foucault 1983: 208). In the prenatal clinic, professionals categorise the objects and subjects of their inter-actions using discourse such as 'foetus/baby' and 'parent'. Such categorisation practices allow people to establish schemes of meaning and make meaning and order so that certain things seem 'natural'. Thus, exploring how professionals find consistency and stability in categories of certain clinical duties and people/things (e.g. professionals, parents, foetuses) reveals how they come to construct the social order of the clinic.

Agreeing with Foucault that discourse is never limited to 'words' or people alone, another key feature of this research is a focus on materials and how power relations are transmitted via artefacts and spaces in different settings. As Latour (1991: 103) claims, we can only account for power 'once the nonhuman are woven into the social fabric'. In short, I recognise how power becomes transmitted via materials and the spatial organisation of Freymarsh and Springtown. The value of attending to the social meanings of materials has a long history in science and technology studies. Scientific theories and conclusions are never made in a vacuum. Many human and nonhuman resources share the scene and lead to stabilising an order; they are drawn on, implicitly and explicitly, to formulate knowledge (Latour 1987; Law 1991). It is in this relational materialism – how assemblages of people, things, space, and talk work together in performing and ordering the social – that neither the technical nor social vision will come into being without the other. Although I would not define my research as an actor-network theory study, I do treat materials and space seriously rather than as 'second class citizens' (Law 1991: 6). By thinking socio-technically and pressing how situated encounters are both social and technical accomplishments, I view the prenatal clinic as a site of 'simultaneous and imbricated material and discursive construction' (Rapp 2000: 194). Making the materials of Freymarsh and Springtown – the ultrasound machines, medical records, furniture, and so forth – explicit and central, rather than implicit and marginal, is of paramount importance for grasping everyday life in the clinic. Materials, indeed, make the clinic 'durable' (Latour 1991).

Finally, as clarified, I am interested in the 'accounts' of professionals with regard to Down's syndrome screening. Cross-checking such accounts with observations of professionals' everyday practices means I am able to reveal the discrepancies between what they *do* and what they *say*. I do not treat such inconsistencies as 'infractions' (Goffman 1971) or 'breaches' (Garfinkel 1967) or, at worst, as untruths. Rather, I view them as instances of 'motility', referring to how people or things are moved in different spaces of discourse (Latimer 2013; Latimer and Munro 2006). The concept of motility is significant for this book. What is made important or unimportant, present or absent, changes from moment to moment. Thus, I capture how such shifts emerge in the everyday work of professionals. I also intermesh this with the concept of 'disposal' (Latimer 1997; Munro 2001). I understand disposal as the means through which professionals engage in ordering work, that is, how they place, displace, and replace certain persons, ideas, or things. I relate the concept of disposal to how professionals classify certain tasks (i.e. Down's syndrome screening) in everyday practice, in relation to identity-work and membership, and how they erect an understanding of certain subjects. Berg (1992) claims that within medicine, physicians construct medical disposals; they dissemble patients into traits so that they can be classified and subsequently disposed of. Medical criteria and disposal options are not 'givens' which lead a physician towards a certain decision. Rather, the physician actively moulds and reconstructs the patient so that their problems are solvable. In this study, I explore how professionals – with reference to classificatory systems – 'detach from' (Latimer 2004) and transform certain tasks and people in particular ways.

In outlining the key theoretical undercurrents which inform my approach, I underline the virtues found in practising theoretical pluralism in opposition to developing a 'grand narrative' (Law 1991). Whilst specific theories are not always explicitly cited or deployed as a framework for interpreting data, they are deeply embedded in the fabric of my arguments. Martin (2010: 24) claims that attending to the interplay of practices, discourses, and materials 'provides a window into the coming-into-being of novel scientific facts and entities'. I detract focus from the *novel* by analysing the old frontier of Down's syndrome screening (it is often popular to analyse new reproductive technologies rather than those deeply embedded in clinical practice) yet, like Martin, I suggest that the mundane relations between practices, discourses, and materials are essential in contemplating the everyday politics of prenatal care, and particularly of prenatal screening practices. Interested in the content of medical action, I reveal how Down's syndrome screening is 'done', how local matters are important for grasping the life of the clinic as a site of bio-politics (Latimer and Thomas 2015), and how reproductive politics are worked through in the familiar scenes of everyday affairs and in the practical accomplishments of professionals. In so doing, I resist subscribing to the notion that certain frameworks or categories are *givens* that defy interpretation. Rather than affording Down's syndrome screening and the condition itself some unquestioned ontological status, I view them as 'things' continually assembled and negotiated in the talk, relations, and practices of professionals.

The study

The research took place between 2011 and 2012 in two locations: (1) Freymarsh, a large NHS teaching hospital in a metropolitan area; and (2) Springtown, a privately funded fertility clinic located in an affluent area. Two clarifications are provided here. First, I will not draw on data exclusively concerning parents-to-be. The views of parents-to-be, with respect to Down's syndrome screening, are undeniably valuable and a key locus of enquiry that has flooded the sociological, psychological, and medical literature. Although I explore their interactions with professionals, I resist regurgitating earlier arguments. Instead, I follow the (much-neglected) professionals, as creatures of habit and bearers of culture, through their worlds. I reveal how their schedules, practices, discourses, and interactions with parents-to-be, colleagues, and materials come to accomplish, intensify, and disturb orders and routines. This study, as such, chimes with earlier hospital ethnographies and classic interactionist work on the clinic showing how professionals and others 'do' medical work in daily interactions, practices, and routines (Atkinson 1995; Bosk 1979; 1992; Davis 1982; Latimer 2000; Silverman 1981; 1987; Strong 1979). By recognising the hospital as a privileged environment for studying the dramatisation of routines, I describe who does what, where, how, to whom, to what end, and its consequences for those involved. I illuminate how ideas around screening for Down's syndrome in the world of healthcare, as a political and contested site, are produced and made sense of from within social, cultural, and medical repertoires – a dynamic frequently missing in current analyses of Down's syndrome screening. Second, whilst I draw upon my observations of two clinics, this is not a comparative study. Whilst the sites differed in some respects, many of the issues raised in this book were evident in Freymarsh *and* Springtown. Furthermore, many professionals at Springtown also worked at Freymarsh. Whilst comparisons did emerge, these would not hold ground as a book. Rather, I draw on fieldwork in each setting to make wider claims about Down's syndrome screening and how it intersects with 'the politics of reproduction' (Ginsburg and Rapp 1991).

The research setting

By limiting my focus to two institutions, I had ample time and space to formulate deep, rich insights into the social life of each setting. I now describe the three places where I spent most of my fieldwork.

Freymarsh antenatal department (FAD)

Freymarsh is an NHS institution. Alignments to notions of welfare are considered one of the key features of NHS hospitals in the UK since services are essentially free at the point of delivery. Yet NHS hospital services are increasingly inscribed with a political and economic rationality and confined by bureaucratic principles designed to achieve goals as precisely, unambiguously, and efficiently as possible. Rather than attempting to critique this rationalisation of the NHS, however, I reveal how such principles are enacted in everyday interactions and the effect this has on both professionals and parents-to-be in prenatal care (more on this later).

Freymarsh's antenatal department (FAD) is located near other pregnancy-related departments such as the delivery suite, maternity department, early pregnancy assessment, and gynaecology department. On arrival at the FAD, parents-to-be are greeted by a large open area beginning either with a small cafe to the right or a reception desk directly meeting one's gaze (depending on which entrance is used). The usually loud and hectic room – professionals can experience slack periods with alternating episodes of chaos – contains many chairs frequently filled with mothers-to-be who are either alone or accompanied by partners and/or children. The walls are relatively drab excepting two television screens displaying BabyTV, a channel played in prenatal waiting rooms nationwide. The channel advertises itself as sharing relevant information to help parents-to-be 'make informed decisions for the health, welfare, safety and happiness of both themselves and their future baby'. Advertised with the tag line 'keeping you informed', the channel includes adverts for baby items (e.g. cots), advice (e.g. bullet-pointed guidance for reducing the risk of cot death), safety advice (e.g. scalds), and video clips of breastfeeding. Near this waiting room are nine other rooms: a staff office, cloakroom, medical supplies closet, room for staff meetings, and five consultation rooms (three of which contain ultrasound equipment). FAD employs around fifteen to twenty midwives (see: Table 0.1), three maternity care assistants (Jennifer, Michelle, Rosie), and three members of administrative staff (Pauline, Whitney, Yvonne). Approximately eight to ten midwives, two maternity care assistants, and two administrative staff work each shift.

Freymarsh foetal medicine department (FMD)

Freymarsh's foetal medicine department (FMD) is located a short walk from FAD. A relatively small department, FMD is a referral unit providing a service to the local/regional population for those with a previous history of maternal/foetal conditions or whose current pregnancy is deemed to require intervention. It has close working links with many departments including FAD, genetics, radiology, cardiology, and neonatology. Parents-to-be consenting to Down's syndrome screening are referred here if they opt for diagnostic testing following a 'higher-risk' result (an explanation of what this means is provided in Chapter 2) and/or choose to terminate a pregnancy following a diagnosis. When attending FMD, parents-to-be enter a small waiting room located outside of six other rooms: two consultation rooms (where parents-to-be receive information about their pregnancy and consent is gained if a procedure is undertaken), an ultrasound scanning room (where most procedures take place), a rarely used small office with space for one person, a small consultation room now used as storage space, and the largest office where most professionals gather. One wall in the waiting room is adorned with a large picture display of recently born babies with cleft lip/palate and other conditions (the 'cleft board'). FMD is run by two consultants (Dr Karman and Dr Cassidy) and employs three head midwives (Elena, Francine, Joanna), four midwives (Emma, Lois, Nancy, Robyn), and one receptionist (Fiona).[11] One consultant, one head midwife, two midwives, and one receptionist typically work each shift.

Springtown antenatal department (SAD)

Springtown is a privately funded fertility clinic located in a grand building situated in an affluent area. It provides a service for pregnant and non-pregnant women including those concerned about miscarriage, fertility, sexual health, and ovarian cancer. Parents-to-be attending the antenatal department (SAD) can pay for ultrasound scans including early pregnancy scans, nuchal translucency[12] scans, growth/wellbeing scans, and cardiac scans.[13] Diagnostic procedures (amniocentesis, CVS) can be offered although parents-to-be are recommended, if consenting to this test, to undertake it in the NHS where no payment is required. On entry, clients approach the reception desk and are directed to the waiting area containing one television, ten chairs, and a water cooler. SAD is a small space with plain corridor walls adorned with pictures of both unborn and newborn babies. SAD contains three rooms: an ultrasound room, a bloods room, and a consultation room. The ultrasound room, where many parents-to-be spend most of their time in SAD, is a dark space containing a large ultrasound machine, two chairs, a large television monitor, a computer, and two photographs of water babies.[14] The ultrasound machine consists of a transducer, a central processing unit, a monitor, and a keyboard. The machine displays body tissue in shades of grey according to its density and allows for the visualisation of a foetus and the measurement of its anatomy (for gestational age). Among other factors, the gestation time determined here is used for medical decision-making. SAD employs two consultants (Dr Finley and Dr Karman), five sonographers (Esther, Heather, Lisa, Olivia, Sophie), four nurses (Francine, Isobel, Keri, Victoria), and four administrative staff (Bethan, Dominique, Hannah, Juliana). One consultant or sonographer and one nurse will work each shift. At least two administrative staff work a shift in an office located near SAD. Most Springtown professionals also work in Freymarsh. For the most part, they undertake the same roles in Springtown as in Freymarsh, even if bestowed with different titles. For example, Francine – a 'nurse' in SAD and 'head midwife' in FMD – performs similar roles at each institution (see Table 0.1).

There are two clear reasons why parents-to-be choose to pursue Down's syndrome screening in Springtown (the privately funded clinic) rather than Freymarsh (the NHS institution). First, Down's syndrome screening in Springtown is heralded as being more 'clinically accurate' (i.e. better detection rate and lower false-positive rate) than Freymarsh. Second, parents-to-be may want to have Down's syndrome screening and receive a result as early as possible, with Springtown offering the procedure earlier in the pregnancy than in Freymarsh. I am clearly simplifying complex decision-making processes here. There are likely to be several other justifications for consenting to Down's syndrome screening in a privately funded clinic, such as parents-to-be worrying after previous pregnancy complications and/or wanting to pursue more 'personable' care. However, earlier and more accurate tests may be why parents-to-be choose to screen for Down's syndrome in Springtown rather than Freymarsh.

Book outline

This book, hereafter, is separated into six chapters. Following this introduction, Chapter 2 contains a brief socio-historical narrative of Down's syndrome screening and how the condition has intersected with scientific and medical worlds since the nineteenth century. This socio-history continues with an outline of Down's syndrome screening in recent years and its current use in Freymarsh and Springtown. Chapter 3 begins with the presentation of data. In this chapter, I explore how Down's syndrome screening is organised in the everyday practices of Freymarsh and Springtown (though I mostly focus on Freymarsh) and how it becomes 'downgraded' in various ways. First, I capture how the task of 'doing' screening, at least initially, is relegated from consultants to midwives (Freymarsh) and sonographers (Springtown). In what follows, I explain how professionals implicitly and explicitly define Down's syndrome screening, in both the frontstage and backstage of the clinic, as a routine affair. Finally, I explore how midwives and sonographers classify screening consultations as a repetitive and valueless task, with other duties being prioritised and preferred for professional identity-work. Since screening – constituting what I call 'hands-off work' – is not aligned with and is not invested with value, it becomes downgraded as a routine matter.

Chapter 4 explores the conduct of care and how the naturalisation/routinisation of Down's syndrome screening as a 'normal' part of pregnancy is accomplished in everyday affairs in two different ways. First, professionals 'dispose' of Down's syndrome screening by using the entwining rhetoric of 'informed choice' and 'non-directive care' to allocate full responsibility for this procedure to parents-to-be. This rhetoric is productive in that it allows professionals to perform 'good care' by giving clinically accurate information devoid of personal bias, avoid decision-making accountability by assuming distance, and suppress their own concerns and unease with screening for Down's syndrome. Second, screening is downgraded by the promotion of the 'social' dimensions of ultrasound scans over 'medical' dimensions (i.e. to detect potential medical issues with a foetus). Professionals merge medical information with a consumer-friendly performance which, in turn, trivialises screening and downgrades its value as a medical practice. Such moves shape engaging with screening as normal and expected conduct for parents-to-be; by being made ordinary, its universal presence in prenatal care becomes unquestioned.

Chapter 5 explores how Down's syndrome itself is constituted in screening consultations and prenatal care more generally. Professionals are frequently ambivalent toward, and express anxieties about, Down's syndrome screening and are frequently positive about the condition. Yet during screening consultations, such principles and interpretations become absent. Indeed, Down's syndrome is talked *around* rather than being talked *about* or *through*. As such, it becomes subsumed by the broader, universalising, and more negative discourse of 'risk', 'problem', or 'abnormality'. The negative portrayal of Down's syndrome remains intact and, therefore, contributes to the persistence of screening in prenatal care. In Chapter 6, the last chapter that presents data, I examine how screening brings cultural ideals around perfection close to hand. This positions parents-to-be, and especially mothers-to-be at an 'advanced maternal age', as exclusively – and morally – accountable for reproductive choices and out-comes. In what follows, I show how the notion that foetuses are 'perfectible' (Ivry 2006: 459) also corresponds to the constitution of Down's syndrome in prenatal care. Extending the claims of Chapter 5, I show how the ambiguity surrounding Down's syndrome – as a condition that is 'compatible with life' (clinically defined) but also that constitutes a legal reason for offering a termi-nation of pregnancy – means that the unborn entity with, or suspected as having, Down's syndrome is often classified by professionals as a 'foetus' as opposed to a 'baby'. It is in the categorical work of professionals that a 'foetus' with Down's syndrome is disposed of in the clinic.

Chapter 7 concludes the book by further contemplating how Down's syn-drome screening plays a central role in reproductive politics, it simultaneously invigorating parental expectations and providing a commentary on what lives are valued (or not). In conjunction with earlier chapters outlining how Down's syndrome screening is downgraded, I argue that screening persists through the (often subtle) constitution of Down's syndrome, and arguably disability more generally, as a negative pregnancy outcome, meaning that certain ways of *being* in the world become stigmatised, denied, silenced, and/or effaced. Thus, I show how prenatal technologies, rather than being perceived solely as a positive knowledge practice for medical and social advancement, reproduce the idealised (unborn) body to collude in a form of exclusion. I offer some recommendations for future prenatal practice, particularly in the context of non-invasive prenatal testing (NIPT) which, at the time of writing, has entered the prenatal arena. However, whilst suggestions are proposed, I do not offer any political or moral disclaimers about Down's syndrome screening. The intention of the book, therefore, is not 'to present a lullaby but merely to sneak in and watch the way the people snore' (Goffman 1974: 74).

Taken together, the chapters tell a story of both extraordinary drama and ordinary routine. By providing thick descriptions of often slim encounters and answering Han's (2013) call for analysing the humdrum and banal aspects of pregnancy, I document a select crosscut of professionals' worlds with important implications for our conceptions of pregnancy, parenthood, disability, and ab/normality, to name a few. Throughout the book, I see Down's syndrome screening not as a patient-centred, individual transaction between profes-sionals and parents-to-be but, rather, as a complicated and collective social and cultural concern that extends beyond the clinic walls and powerfully shapes the makeup of contemporary society. It is challenging to make claims about a specific (and widespread) medical practice on the basis of a single study. However, my analysis in this book answers broad universal questions about the place of Down's syndrome in reproductive politics. I am optimistic that my arguments translate elsewhere and, so, provide stimulus or at least some scaffolding for scholars to critically explore other forms of screening in different contexts.

Notes

1 The term 'compatible with life' is synonymous with 'viable' to refer to babies that are likely to survive childbirth and to have a 'quality of life' that is not 'life-limiting' (using the discourse of UK medicine). The term 'compatible with life' is used throughout this book as it is the term most commonly used by professionals in the study.

2 Edward's syndrome (Trisomy 18) and Patau syndrome (Trisomy 13) are chromosomal conditions. Whilst Edward's syndrome occurs in three of every 10,000 live births, Patau syndrome affects two of every 10,000 live births. Both conditions are caused by an extra copy of a chromosome (chromosome 18 for Edward's, and chromosome 13 for Patau) in each cell and manifest in three forms: complete, mosaic, and partial. According to NHS FASP (2012), both conditions are fatal. The conditions are associated with intellectual disability and physiological impairment. Babies with partial and mosaic Trisomy 18 or Trisomy 13 may survive to adulthood but this is reported as being rare.

3 The term 'parents-to-be' is my own. Professionals in this study frequently use 'lady', 'woman', 'parent', or 'mum' to describe such people. I have used my own term for consistency. I also use the terms 'mother-to-be' and 'father-to-be' when appropriate.

4 The terms 'foetus' and 'baby' are inherently problematic. Whilst anti-abortionists use the words 'baby' or 'unborn child', feminists will likely opt for 'foetus' to avoid giving a foetus human status (Williams 2002). This is complicated by pregnant women themselves often not using the term foetus. In this book, I mostly assume the term foetus but I stress that this is not indicative of an explicit moral or ethical commitment. Rather, it is used since it is the language employed, for the most part, in the domain that I studied: prenatal medicine. That said, as will be shown throughout this book, and particularly in Chapter 6, the use of the terms 'foetus' and 'baby' can shift at different moments.

5 Down's syndrome screening uptake statistics in Scotland or Northern Ireland could not be identified. However, the National Services Division (2011) claims 34,768 mothers-to-be in Scotland were screened for Down's syndrome in 2010/2011. It is worth noting, though, that such statistics do not represent all procedures in Scotland as it is limited to those collected by nationally designated laboratories. In addition, interviews conducted with 666 mothers-to-be across two hospitals in Northern Ireland suggests a lower acceptance rate (26% and 28%) than reported in England and Wales (McNeill et al. 2009). I suspect that this corresponds to termination of a pregnancy for Down's syndrome being illegal in Northern Ireland (at the time of writing).

6 The low uptake rates in Japan are perhaps attributable to a lack of information on prenatal diagnosis and to abortion not being legally permitted for 'foetal abnormalities' (Nishiyama et al. 2013).

7 The tag of Down's syndrome screening is confusing. This is because prenatal screening, as it currently stands, also involves screening and producing risk factors

for two other conditions: Patau syndrome and Edward's syndrome. In addition, it is worth reiterating that a screening test does not produce a diagnosis but rather provides parents-to-be with information about the chance of their foetus having a condition. In contrast, a diagnostic test can establish the presence or absence of a condition in a foetus, though it should be noted that diagnostic tests are not 100% accurate and are susceptible to human error.

8 Although I provide a short summary of such work here, I have produced a more extensive examination of current literature on the experiences of parents and professionals when screening for Down's syndrome – as well as the common justifications for parents consenting, or not, to screening – elsewhere (Thomas 2014). Reid et al. (2009) and Skirton and Barr (2007) also offer excellent summaries of pregnant women's decision-making processes relating to Down's syndrome screening.

9 I recognise that the term 'disability' is widely contested (Davis 1995; Shakespeare 2006), particularly relating to its relationship with 'impairment'. Throughout this book, I mostly employ the term 'disability' because this is used most frequently by Freymarsh and Springtown professionals when referring to the loss of physiological or psychological function. I am fully aware that this may reflect the 'medical', rather than the 'social', model of disability (Oliver 1990) but I ask for some forbearance here. I also do not intend to debate the social and medical models of disability as much ink has already been spilled over this particular topic.

10 There is a body of literature that identifies how screening more generally – that is, not limited to Down's syndrome screening – is both a social and medical intervention that reproduces certain identities, hierarchies, responsibilities, and values (Armstrong and Eborall 2012; Boardman 2010; Cox and McKellin 1999; Lock et al. 2007; Timmermans and Buchbinder 2013).

11 Professionals from other departments such as cardiology, radiology, or neuroscience are called upon to help with certain cases. In this book, only four such professionals are cited: (1) Annie, a sonographer; (2) Jodi, a cardiac physiologist; (3) Roxanne, a sonographer; (4) Dr Torres, a cardiologist. They are cited as 'Annie (FMD sonographer)', 'Jodi (FMD cardiac physiologist)', 'Roxanne (FMD sonographer)', and 'Dr Torres (FMD cardiologist)'.

12 A nuchal translucency is the fluid thickness in the nape of the foetal neck. Enlarged fluid is associated with chromosomal conditions, such as Down's syndrome.

13 A cardiac scan involves a sonographer, via an ultrasound scan, examining the two outflow tracts and four chambers of the foetal heart. In Springtown, the scan is offered at around twenty-four weeks into a pregnancy.

14 The pictures show a young father smiling and holding his newborn child. Both are photographed underwater. Lisa (SAD sonographer) explains that newborn babies have a natural diving reflex and so avoid inhaling water into their lungs.

Bibliography

Alderson, P. 2001. Down's syndrome: cost, quality and value of life. *Social Science and Medicine* 53(5), pp. 627–638.

Anderson, G. 1999. Nondirectiveness in prenatal genetics: patients read between the lines. *Nursing Ethics* 6(2), pp. 126–136.

Armstrong, N. and Eborall, H. 2012. The sociology of medical screening: past, present and future. *Sociology of Health and Illness* 34(2), pp. 161–176.

Atkinson, P. 1995. *Medical Talk and Medical Work: The Liturgy of the Clinic*. Thousand Oaks, CA: Sage.

Aune, I. and Möller, A. 2012. 'I want choice, but I don't want to decide': a qualitative study of pregnant women's experiences regarding early ultrasound risk assessment for chromosomal anomalies. *Midwifery* 28(1), pp. 14–23.

Baillie, C., Smith, J., Hewisin, J. and Mason, G. 2000. Ultrasound screening for chromosomal abnormality: women's reactions to false positive results. *British Journal of Health Psychology* 5(4), pp. 377–394.

Berg, M. 1992. The construction of medical disposals: medical sociology and medical problem solving in clinical practice. *Sociology of Health and Illness* 14(2), pp. 151–180.

Bérubé, M. 1996. *Life As We Know It: A Father, a Family, and an Exceptional Child*. New York: Pantheon Books.

Boardman, F.K. 2010. *The Role of Experiential Knowledge in the Reproductive Decision Making of Families Genetically At Risk: The Case of Spinal Muscular Atrophy*. Unpublished Ph.D. Thesis, University of Warwick.

Bosk, C.L. 1979. *Forgive and Remember: Managing Medical Failure*. Chicago: University of Chicago Press.

Bosk, C.L. 1992. *All God's Mistakes: Genetic Counseling in a Pediatric Hospital*. Chicago: University of Chicago Press.

Boyd, P.A., DeVigan, C., Khoshnood, B., Loane, M., Garne, E., Dolk, H. and the EUROCAT Working Group. 2008. Survey of prenatal screening policies in Europe for structural malformations and chromosome anomalies, and their impact on detection and termination rates for neural tube defects and Down's syndrome. *BJOG: An International Journal of Obstetrics and Gynaecology* 115(6), pp. 689–696.

Browner, C.H. and Preloran, H.M. 1999. Male partners' role in Latinas' amniocentesis decisions. *Journal of Genetic Counselling* 8(2), pp. 85–108.

Browner, C.H., Preloran, H.M. and Press, N. 1996. The effects of ethnicity, education and an informational video on pregnant women's knowledge and decisions about a prenatal diagnostic screening test. *Patient Education and Counselling* 27(2), pp. 135–146.

Bryant, L.D., Green, J.M. and Hewison, J.D. 2006. Understanding of Down's syndrome: a Q methodological investigation. *Social Science and Medicine* 63(5), pp. 1188–1200.

Buckley, F. and Buckley, S.J. 2008. Wrongful deaths and rightful lives: screening for Down syndrome. *Down Syndrome Research and Practice* 12(2), pp. 79–86.

Burton-Jeangros, C., Cavalli, S., Gouilhers, S. and Hammer, R. 2013. Between tolerable uncertainty and unacceptable risks: how health professionals and pregnant women think about the probabilities generated by prenatal screening. *Health, Risk and Society* 15(2), pp. 144–161.

CARIS. 2012. *CARIS Review 2012*. Swansea: Public Health Wales.

Chiang, H.H., Chao, Y.M. and Yuh, Y.S. 2006. Informed choice of pregnant women in prenatal screening tests for Down's syndrome. *Journal of Medical Ethics* 32(5), pp. 273–277.

Collins, V.R., Muggli, E.E., Riley, M., Dip, G., Palma, S. and Halliday, J.L. 2008. Is Down syndrome a disappearing birth defect? *The Journal of Paediatrics* 152(1), pp. 20–24.

Cowan, R.S. 1994. Women's roles in the history of amniocentesis and chorionic villi sampling. In: Rothenberg, K. and Thomson, E. eds. *Women and Prenatal Testing: Facing the Challenges of Genetic Technology*. Columbus: Ohio State University Press, pp. 35–48.

Cox, S.M. and McKellin, W. 1999. 'There's this thing in our family': predictive testing and the construction of risk for Huntington disease. *Sociology of Health and Illness* 21(5), pp. 622–646.

Crang-Svalenius, E., Dykes, A.K. and Jorgensen, C. 1998. Factors influencing informed choice of prenatal diagnosis: women's feelings and attitudes. *Fetal Diagnosis and Therapy* 13(1), pp. 53–61.

Davis, A.G. 1982. *Children in Clinics: A Sociological Analysis of Medical Work with Children*. London: Tavistock Publications.

Davis, L.J. 1995. *Enforcing Normalcy: Disability, Deafness, and the Body*. London: Verso.

Draper, J. 2002. 'It was a real good show': the ultrasound scan, fathers and the power of visual knowledge. *Sociology of Health and Illness* 24(6), pp. 771–795.

Ekelin, M. and Crang-Svalenius, E. 2004. Midwives' attitudes to and knowledge about a newly introduced fetal screening method. *Scandinavian Journal of Caring Sciences* 18(3), pp. 287–293.

Farsides, B., Williams, C. and Alderson, P. 2004. Aiming towards 'moral equilibrium': health care professionals' views on working within the morally contested field of antenatal screening. *Journal of Medical Ethics* 30(5), pp. 505–509.

Foucault, M. 1972. *The Archaeology of Knowledge*. London: Routledge.

Foucault, M. 1973. *The Birth of the Clinic: An Archaeology of Medical Perception*. London: Tavistock Publications.

Foucault, M. 1980. *Power/Knowledge*. New York: Pantheon.

Foucault, M. 1983. The subject and power. In: Dreyfus, H.L. and Rabinow, P. eds. *Michael Foucault: Beyond Structuralism and Hermeneutics*. Chicago: University of Chicago Press, pp. 208–226.

Franklin, S. and Roberts, C. 2006. *Born and Made: An Ethnography of Preimplantation Genetic Diagnosis*. Princeton, NJ: Princeton University Press.

Gammeltoft, T.M. and Nguyén, H.T.T. 2007. Fetal conditions and fatal decisions: ethical dilemmas in ultrasound screening in Vietnam. *Social Science and Medicine* 64 (11), pp. 2248–2259.

Gammons, S., Sooben, R.D. and Heslam, S. 2010. Support and information about Down's syndrome. *British Journal of Midwifery* 18(11), pp. 700–708.

García, E., Timmermans, D.R.M. and van Leeuwen, E. 2008. The impact of ethical beliefs on decisions about prenatal screening tests: searching for justification. *Social Science and Medicine* 66(3), pp. 753–764.

Garfinkel, H. 1967. *Studies in Ethnomethodology*. Englewood Cliffs, NJ: Prentice-Hall.

Getz, L. and Kirkengen, A.L. 2003. Ultrasound screening in pregnancy: advancing technology, soft markers for foetal chromosomal aberrations, and unacknowledged ethical dilemmas. *Social Science and Medicine* 56(10), pp. 2045–2057.

Ginsburg, F.D. and Rapp, R. 1991. The politics of reproduction. *Annual Review of Anthropology* 20, pp. 311–343.

Goffman, E. 1959. *The Presentation of Self in Everyday Life*. London: Allen Lane.

Goffman, E. 1971. *Relations in Public: Microstudies of the Public Order*. London: Allen Lane.

Goffman, E. 1974. *Frame Analysis: An Essay on the Organization of Experience*. Cambridge: Harvard University Press.

Goffman, E. 1983. The interaction order. *American Sociological Review* 48(1), pp. 1–17.

Gottfreðsdóttir, H., Björnsdóttir, K. and Sandall, J. 2009. 'This is just what you do when you are pregnant': a qualitative study of prospective parents in Iceland who accept nuchal translucency screening. *Midwifery* 25(6), pp. 711–720.

Green, J.M. and Statham, H. 1996. Psychosocial aspects of prenatal screening and diagnosis. In: Marteau, T.M. and Richards, M. eds. *The Troubled Helix: Social and Psychological Implications of the New Human Genetics*. New York: Cambridge University Press, pp. 140–163.

Han, S. 2013. *Pregnancy in Practice: Expectation and Experience in the Contemporary US*. Oxford: Berghahn Books.

Hey, M. and Hurst, K. 2003. Antenatal screening: why do women refuse? *RCM Midwives Journal* 6(5), pp. 216–220.

Heyman, B., Hundy, G., Sandall, J., Spencer, K., Williams, C., Grellier, R. and Pitson, L. 2006. On being at higher risk: a qualitative study of prenatal screening for chromosomal anomalies. *Social Science and Medicine* 62(10), pp. 2360–2372.

Hunt, L., de Voogd, K.B. and Castañeda, H. 2005. The routine and the traumatic in prenatal genetic diagnosis: does clinical information inform patient decision-making? *Patient Education and Counselling* 56(3), pp. 302–312.

Ivry, T. 2006. At the backstage of prenatal care: Japanese ob-gyns negotiating prenatal diagnosis. *Medical Anthropology Quarterly* 20(4), pp. 441–468.

Ivry, T. 2009. The ultrasonic picture show and the politics of threatened life. *Medical Anthropology Quarterly* 23(3), pp. 189–211.

Jaques, A.M., Bell, R.J., Watson, L. and Halliday, J.L. 2004. People who influence women's decisions and preferred sources of information about prenatal testing for birth defects. *Australian and New Zealand Journal of Obstetrics and Gynaecology* 44(3), pp. 233–238.

Kaiser, A.S., Ferris, L.E., Katz, R., Pastuszak, A., Llewellyn-Thomas, H., Johnson, J.A. and Shaw, B.F. 2004. Psychological responses to prenatal NTS counselling and the uptake of invasive testing in women of advanced maternal age. *Patient Education and Counselling* 54(1), pp. 45–53.

Latimer, J.E. 1997. Giving patients a future: the constituting of classes in an acute medical unit. *Sociology of Health and Illness* 19(2), pp. 160–185.

Latimer, J.E. 2000. *The Conduct of Care: Understanding Nursing Practice*. Oxford: Blackwell Science.

Latimer, J.E. 2004. Commanding materials: (re)legitimating authority in the context of multi-disciplinary work. *Sociology* 38(4), pp. 757–775.

Latimer, J.E. 2007. Diagnosis, dysmorphology, and the family: knowledge, motility, choice. *Medical Anthropology* 26(2), pp. 97–138.

Latimer, J.E. 2013. *The Gene, the Clinic and the Family: Diagnosing Dysmorphology, Reviving Medical Dominance*. London: Routledge.

Latimer, J.E. and Munro, R. 2006. Driving the social. *The Sociological Review* 54(S1), pp. 32–53.

Latimer, J.E. and Thomas, G.M. 2015. In/exclusion in the clinic: Down's syndrome, dysmorphology, and the ethics of everyday medical work. *Sociology* 49(5), pp. 937–954.

Latour, B. 1987. *Science in Action: How To Follow Scientists and Engineers Through Society*. Milton Keynes: Open University Press.

Latour, B. 1991. Technology is society made durable. In: Law, J. ed. *A Sociology of Monsters: Essays on Power, Technology and Domination*. London: Routledge, pp. 103–131.

Law, J. 1991. Introduction: monsters, machines and sociotechnical relations. In: Law, J. ed. *A Sociology of Monsters: Essays on Power, Technology and Domination*. London: Routledge, pp. 1–25.

Lippman, A. 1991. Prenatal genetic testing and screening: constructing needs and reinforcing inequities. *American Journal of Law and Medicine* 17(1–2), pp. 15–50.

Lippman, A. 1994. The genetic construction of prenatal testing: choice, consent, or conformity for women? In: Rothenberg, K. and Thomson, E. eds. *Women and Prenatal Testing: Facing the Challenges of Genetic Technology*. Columbus: Ohio State University Press, pp. 9–34.

Lock, M., Freeman, J., Chilibeck, G., Beveridge, B. and Padolsky, M. 2007. Susceptibility genes and the question of embodied identity. *Medical Anthropology Quarterly* 21(3), pp. 256–276.

Lupton, D. 2013. *The Social Worlds of the Unborn*. Hampshire: Palgrave Macmillan.

Markens, S., Browner, C.H. and Preloran, H.M. 2010. Interrogating the dynamics between power, knowledge and pregnant bodies in amniocentesis decision making. *Sociology of Health and Illness* 32(1), pp. 37–56.

Markens, S., Browner, C.H. and Press, N. 1999. 'Because of the risks': how US pregnant women account for refusing prenatal screening. *Social Science and Medicine* 49(3), pp. 359–369.

Marteau, T.M. 1995. Towards informed decisions about prenatal testing: a review. *Prenatal Diagnosis* 15(13), pp. 1215–1226.

Marteau, T.M., Kidd, J., Michie, S., Cook, R., Johnston, M. and Shaw, R. 1993. Anxiety, knowledge and satisfaction in women receiving false positive results on routine prenatal screening: a randomised controlled trial. *Journal of Psychosomatic Obstetrics and Gynaecology* 14(3), pp. 185–196.

Martin, A. 2010. Microchimerism in the mother(land): blurring the borders of body and nation. *Body and Society* 16(3), pp. 23–50.

McCourt, C. 2006. Supporting choice and control? Communication and interaction between midwives and women at the antenatal booking visit. *Social Science and Medicine* 62(6), pp. 1307–1318.

McNeill, J., Alderdice, F., Rowe, R., Martin, D. and Dornan, J.C. 2009. Down's syndrome screening in Northern Ireland: women's reasons for accepting or declining serum testing. *Evidence Based Midwifery* 7(3), pp. 76–83.

Mitchell, L.M. and Georges, E. 1998. Baby's first picture. In: Davis-Floyd, R. and Dumit, R. eds. *Cyborg Babies: From Techno-Sex to Techno-Tots*. New York: Routledge, pp. 105–124.

Morris, J.K. and Springett, A. 2014. *The National Down Syndrome Cytogenetic Register for England and Wales: 2013 Annual Report*. London: Wolfson Institute of Preventive Medicine.

Munro, R. 2001. Disposal of the body: upending postmodernism. *Ephemera* 1(2), pp. 108–130.

National Services Division. 2011. *National Services Division Annual Report 2010/11*. Edinburgh: National Services Division.

Natoli, J.L., Ackerman, D.L., McDermott, S. and Edwards, J.G. 2012. Prenatal diagnosis of Down syndrome: a systematic review of termination rates (1995–2011). *Prenatal Diagnosis* 32(2), pp. 142–153.

NHS FASP. 2012. *NHS Fetal Anomaly Screening Programme: Annual Report 2011–2012*. University of Exeter: NHS Fetal Anomaly Screening Programme.

Nishiyama, M., Sawai, H. and Kosugi, S. 2013. The current state of genetic counselling before and after amniocentesis for foetal karyotyping in Japan: a survey of obstetric hospital clients of a prenatal testing laboratory. *Journal of Genetic Counselling* 22(6), pp. 795–804.

Oliver, M. 1990. *The Politics of Disablement*. Basingstoke: Macmillan.

ONS. 2011. *Statistical Bulletin: Live Births in England and Wales by Characteristics of Mother 1, 2011*. Newport: Office for National Statistics.

Parens, E. and Asch, A. 2000. *Prenatal Testing and Disability Rights*. Washington, DC: Georgetown University Press.

Pilnick, A. 2004. 'It's just one of the best tests that we've got at the moment': the presentation of nuchal translucency screening for fetal abnormality in pregnancy. *Discourse and Society* 15(4), pp. 451–465.

Pilnick, A. 2008. 'It's something for you both to think about': choice and decision-making in nuchal translucency screening for Down's syndrome. *Sociology of Health and Illness* 30(4), pp. 511–530.

Pilnick, A., Fraser, D.M. and James, D.K. 2004. Presenting and discussing nuchal translucency screening for fetal abnormality in the UK. *Midwifery* 20(1), pp. 82–93.

Pilnick, A. and Zayts, O. 2012. 'Let's have it tested first': choice and circumstances in decision-making following positive antenatal screening in Hong Kong. *Sociology of Health and Illness* 34(2), pp. 266–282.

Press, N. and Browner, C.H. 1997. Why women say yes to prenatal diagnosis. *Social Science and Medicine* 45(7), pp. 979–989.

Rapp, R. 2000. *Testing Women, Testing the Fetus: The Social Impact of Amniocentesis in America*. London: Routledge.

Reed, K. 2012. *Gender and Genetics: Sociology of the Prenatal*. London: Routledge.

Reid, B., Sinclair, M., Barr, O., Dobbs, F. and Crealey, G. 2009. A meta-synthesis of pregnant women's decision-making processes with regard to antenatal screening for Down syndrome. *Social Science and Medicine* 69(11), pp. 1561–1573.

Remennick, L. 2006. The quest for the perfect baby: why do Israeli women seek prenatal genetic testing? *Sociology of Health and Illness* 28(1), pp. 21–53.

Rothman, B.K. 1986. *The Tentative Pregnancy: Amniocentesis and the Sexual Politics of Motherhood*. London: Pandora.

Rothman, B.K. 1998. *Genetic Maps and Human Imaginations: The Limits of Science in Understanding Who We Are*. New York: Norton.

Samwill, L. 2002. Midwives' knowledge of Down's syndrome screening. *British Journal of Midwifery* 10(4), pp. 247–250.

Santalahti, P., Hemminki, E., Latikka, A.M. and Ryynanen, M. 1998. Women's decision making in prenatal screening. *Social Science and Medicine* 46(8), pp. 1067–1076.

Schwennesen, N. and Koch, L. 2012. Representing and intervening: 'doing' good care in first trimester prenatal knowledge production and decision-making. *Sociology of Health and Illness* 34(2), pp. 282–298.

Scott, S., Hinton-Smith, T., Härmä, V. and Broome, K. 2013. Goffman in the gallery: interactive art and visitor shyness. *Symbolic Interaction* 36(4), pp. 417–438.

Seavilleklein, V. 2009. Challenging the rhetoric of choice in prenatal screening. *Bioethics* 23(1), pp. 68–77.

Shakespeare, T.W. 2006. *Disability Rights and Wrongs*. London: Routledge.

Shakespeare, T.W. 2011. Choices, reasons and feelings: prenatal diagnosis as disability dilemma. *European Journal of Disability Research* 5(1), pp. 37–43.

Silverman, D. 1981. The child as social object: Down's syndrome children in a paediatric cardiology clinic. *Sociology of Health and Illness* 3(3), pp. 254–274.

Silverman, D. 1987. *Communication and Medical Practice: Social Relations in the Clinic*. London: Sage.

Skirton, H. and Barr, O. 2007. Influences on uptake of antenatal screening for Down's syndrome: a review of the literature. *Evidence Based Midwifery* 5(1), pp. 4–9.

Sooben, R.D. 2010. Antenatal testing and the subsequent birth of a child with Down syndrome: a phenomenological study of parents' experiences. *Journal of Intellectual Disabilities* 14(2), pp. 79–94.

Strong, P. 1979. *The Ceremonial Order of the Clinic: Parents, Doctors and Medical Bureaucracies.* Henley-on-Thames: Routledge and Kegan Paul.

Ternby, E., Ingvoldstad, C., Annerén, G. and Axelsson, O. 2015. Midwives and information on prenatal testing with focus on Down syndrome. *Prenatal Diagnosis* 35(12), pp. 1202–1207.

Thomas, G.M. 2014. Prenatal screening for Down's syndrome: parent and healthcare practitioner experiences. *Sociology Compass* 8(6), pp. 837–850.

Timmermans, S. and Buchbinder, M. 2013. *Saving Babies? The Consequences of Newborn Genetic Screening.* Chicago: University of Chicago Press.

Tsouroufli, M. 2011. Routinisation and constraints on informed choice in a one-stop clinic offering first trimester chromosomal antenatal screening for Down's syndrome. *Midwifery* 27(4), pp. 431–436.

van den Berg, M., Timmmermans, D.R., Kleinveld, J.H., García, E., van Vugt, J.M. and van der Wal, G. 2005a. Accepting or declining the offer of prenatal screening for congenital defects: test uptake and women's reasons. *Prenatal Diagnosis* 25(1), pp. 84–90.

van den Berg, M., Timmermans, D.R., ten Kate, L.P., van Vugt, J.M. and van der Wal, G. 2005b. Are pregnant women making informed choices about antenatal screening? *Genetics in Medicine* 7(5), pp. 332–338.

Vassy, C. 2006. From a genetic innovation to mass health programmes: the diffusion of Down's syndrome prenatal screening and diagnostic techniques in France. *Social Science and Medicine* 63(8), pp. 2041–2051.

Vassy, C., Rosman, S., and Rousseau, B. 2014. From policy making to service use: Down's syndrome antenatal screening in England, France and the Netherlands. *Social Science and Medicine* 106, pp. 67–74.

Wasserman, D. and Asch, A. 2006. The uncertain rationale for prenatal disability screening. *American Medical Association Journal of Ethics* 8(1), pp. 53–56.

Williams, C. 2002. Framing the foetus in medical work: rituals and practices. *Social Science and Medicine* 60(9), pp. 2085–2095.

Williams, C. 2006. Dilemmas in fetal medicine: premature application of technology corresponding to women's choice? *Sociology of Health and Illness* 28(1), pp. 1–20.

Williams, C., Alderson, P. and Farsides, B. 2002a. Dilemmas encountered by health practitioners offering nuchal translucency screening: a qualitative case study. *Prenatal Diagnosis* 22(3), pp. 216–220.

Williams, C., Alderson, P. and Farsides, B. 2002b. 'Drawing the line' in prenatal screening and testing: health practitioners' discussions. *Health, Risk and Society* 4(1), pp. 61–75.

Williams, C., Alderson, P. and Farsides, B. 2002c. Is nondirectiveness possible within the context of antenatal screening and testing? *Social Science and Medicine* 54(3), pp. 339–347.

Williams, C., Alderson, P. and Farsides, B. 2002d. Too many choices? Hospital and community staff reflect on the future of prenatal screening. *Social Science and Medicine* 55(5), pp. 743–753.

Williams, C., Alderson, P. and Farsides, B. 2002e. What constitutes 'balanced' information in the practitioners' portrayal of Down's syndrome? *Midwifery* 18(3), pp. 230–237.

Williams, C., Sandall, J., Lewando-Hundt, G., Heyman, B., Spencer, K. and Grellier, R. 2005. Women as moral pioneers? Experiences of first trimester antenatal screening. *Social Science and Medicine* 61(9), pp. 1983–1992.

Zimmerman, D.H. and Pollner, M. 1970. The everyday world as a phenomenon. In: Douglas, J.D. ed. *Understanding Everyday Life: Towards a Reconstruction of Sociological Knowledge*. London: Routledge and Kegan Paul, pp. 80–103.

Chapter 2

A short socio-history

This chapter begins by outlining how Down's syndrome has become the main target of prenatal screening. Starting from the position that one must have a firm grasp of the past to both understand the present and ponder the future, I piece together key moments within the last 200 years, both inside and outside of the UK, that have contributed to Down's syndrome being subjected to the pervasive reproductive gaze. A range of social, technological, scientific, legal, economic, political, and cultural developments have stimulated new research and clinical tools around Down's syndrome and detecting the condition in prenatal care, from the contested to the mundane. What I suggest is that Down's syndrome and its intersection with prenatal care evolved in a gradual and mostly undisputed fashion. To draw upon another example, Casper and Clarke (1998: 255) show how the pap smear became the 'right tool for the job' for cervical cancer screening. Technical manipulation, the automation of record-keeping, the proliferation of health activists, public pressure following high rates of incorrect readings, and the creation of the American Cancer Society, among other trends, created the environment necessary for supporting its development and subsequent diffusion. Similar to Casper and Clarke, I identify how Down's syndrome screening has become a routine process, that is, the 'right tool for the job' in prenatal care. This concise socio-history is loosely chronological but messy and convoluted, reflecting the immense complexity of how the diagnostic category of Down's syndrome and screening for the condition have come into being. I am indebted here to the insights offered by historians (Cowan 1994; Löwy 2014a; 2014b; Wright 2011), healthcare professionals (Nancollas 2012; Reynolds 2010), anthropologists (Rapp 2000), and parents of children with Down's syndrome (Bérubé 1996; Logan 2011).[1]

The making of mongolism

The inception of the category 'mongolism' or 'idiocy' (i.e. what is now referred to as Down's syndrome)[2] seemingly began in 1838 with the publication of Jean-Étienne Dominique Esquirol's *Des Maladies Mentales Considérées Sous les*

Rapports Médical, Hygiènique et Médico-Légal, Volume 1. A psychiatrist by trade, Esquirol described a particular collection of people as 'idiots', roughly translating as those with intellectual and developmental disabilities. This work was developed by his colleague Édouard Séguin, a physician and educationist working with children who had cognitive impairments. Séguin's book, *Traitment Moral, Hygiène et Éducation des Idiots et des Autres Enfants Arriérés* (1846), was dedicated to the diagnosis and treatment of such children, arguing that they could undertake 'moral treatment' to help them to socialise with others and to contribute more effectively to society (mostly through physical labour). However, the formal category of mongolism was more famously developed by English physician John Langdon Down in 1866. Working at the Royal Earlswood Asylum for Idiots, Down ([1866] 1997) was the first person to comprehensively describe a group of people sharing anatomical and behavioural characteristics, a group that he defined as 'mongoloids' given that their facial features were seen as similar to people of Mongolian descent. Although it is reported that the scientific basis of this designation was contested and rejected, the name remained for many years.

Pueschel (2000) offers three reasons for why mongolism was not previously recognised as a clinical entity. First, few physicians before the nineteenth century were interested in children with developmental conditions. Second, the prevalence of many diseases and conditions would have overshadowed mongolism. Nancollas (2012: 46) similarly argues that this lack of recognition may have occurred since people with Down's syndrome, inhabiting a society marked by people with many different conditions and diseases, 'did not particularly stand out'. Third, for Pueschel, only half of women aged above thirty-five survived during this period, arguably resulting in lower amounts of late-aged pregnancies in which women were likely to have a child with mongolism (more on this later). Nonetheless, it is within this time period that mongolism as a diagnostic category was *made*, namely, that it was constituted by social and medical/scientific discourse.[3]

Institutionalisation and eugenics

So how were people with mongolism treated in this period? Some training schools in nineteenth-century Europe (e.g. Germany, Switzerland) and the USA were opened for people with learning disabilities, mongolism included. Institutions dedicated to the treatment and training of such people included the State Asylum for Idiots in New York (1854), the Pennsylvania Training School for Idiotic and Feeble-Minded Children (1852), and the Ohio Asylum for Feebleminded Youth (1857). In the UK, institutions were also established in England, Wales, Scotland, and Ireland in the nineteenth century. Such settings were, in theory, designed to be curative; they were viewed as new and humane sites where people could be treated, trained, and educated by experts. Whilst not offering a cure, and abuse being reported, improvements in the behaviour, physicality, and social competence of people with mongolism were described. *by whom?!*

However, a sudden economic downturn meant no opportunity for employment for those housed in training schools. As such, schools expanded but quickly became asylums that provided basic levels of care for their inhabitants. Such institutions also became colonised by medicine, with doctors and custodians now working inside the premises. This shift was undoubtedly influenced by the Enlightenment period, whereby people with mongolism and other disabilities were recast from marginal medical topics to important test cases for developing scientific knowledge (possible causes for mongolism that were suggested at this time included alcoholic parents, syphilitic infection, tuberculosis, and 'uterine exhaustion'). This meant, however, that rather than being educated and returned to the community, many inhabitants were identified as requiring treatment or a cure. The medicalisation of training schools, in turn, produced systemised prejudices towards people with disabilities, including those with mongolism, as sick and in need of medical management. This reflected a shift in public consciousness from compassion and care to burden and segregation, that is, from education to protecting society from those considered as social undesirables (Wright 2011).

Whilst originally designed under idealistic aspirations of offering asylum, such schools became 'total institutions' (Goffman 1961). People that were seen as a danger to themselves and others were incarcerated and forcibly restrained, meaning that institutions became secure lodgings for the 'strange' and dispossessed. Indeed, social problems such as poverty resulted in many individuals being housed in such institutions (i.e. not solely for people with mongolism). This was a form of 'sequestration' (Giddens 1991: 165), in which the expansion of technical knowledge led to the 'sick and dying' being separated from 'normal' members of society. The sequestration of people with mongolism or other conditions meant that their fate became a technical matter that was handled by medical experts, with inhabitants routinely hidden from public view.

By the early twentieth century, mongolism became the most commonly recognised learning disability, and many people with the syndrome lived their short lives in congested institutions. Wright (2011) suggests that medical professionals interested in mongolism recognised the syndrome as identifiable through a clustering of symptoms such as small stature (Thus Mitchell in 1876), the incurved shape of small fingers (Telford Smith in 1896), and a singular palmar crease (Reginald Langdon Down, son of John Langdon Down, in 1908). However, this interest in the aetiology of the condition, leading to generations of speculation, was supplemented with an anxiety during the Edwardian period, whereby intellectual circles were awash with ideologies of Social Darwinism (Wright 2011). The forced institutionalisation of people with mongolism, indeed, was closely linked to racial and eugenic theory in the early twentieth century. Such concerns around degeneration found their voice in national eugenics movements, with ongoing research being carried out under the shadow of hereditarianism that considered those who were 'feeble-minded' as threatening the welfare of society in general.

Eugenics, a term developed by Galton (1883), represents a theory and practice of improving the genetic quality of humans by pursuing the reproduction of people with desired attributes and reducing the reproduction of those with undesirable attributes. The eugenics movement gained popularity in the early twentieth century in the UK and US scientific and medical community, reflected most profoundly not only by institutionalisation but, also, by enforced sterilisation programmes being carried out globally for people with mongolism and other learning disabilities (Selikowitz 2008). The imperatives of eugenics and the national concerns over the quality of children were also fuelled by other social developments, such as the establishment of elementary education in most countries in the global North. This brought millions of children under state surveillance and, as such, hastened the seclusion of children with mongolism and others seen as feeble-minded into special schools or, more often than not, into asylums. In addition, looming military confrontations further stressed the need for a 'healthy' populace. Many social movements and events, thus, led to state policies of segregation and sterilisation.

The eugenics programme was widely supported in the UK. It did eventually lose scientific credibility but this was not before many people with mongolism had been institutionalised and/or sterilised worldwide in the name of social purity – and before Nazi Germany embraced the strategy. The link between mongolism and eugenics, indeed, was most profoundly shown in the rise of Nazi Germany and the implementation of 'Aktion T4', a euthanasia programme that officially ran from 1939 to 1941 – but was said to continue unofficially thereafter – whereby physicians killed individuals 'judged incurably sick by critical medical examination' (Proctor 1988: 177). People with mongolism, together with people with other conditions, diseases, and/or physical malformations, were characterised in a highly medicalised system as incurably sick (Lifton 1986) and as *untermensch*, a term integral to Nazi racial ideology referring to those deemed to be 'life unworthy of life'. Despite the end of World War II and eugenic policies being rebuffed, people with conditions like mongolism were still being incarcerated in institutions well into the 1970s. In addition, recent historical scholarship reports that state-sanctioned sterilisation and eugenic practices persisted in North America, Europe, and South America for decades after World War II (for statistics, see: Wright 2011: 108).

The French connection: clinical genetics

The rise of eugenics and the institutionalisation of people with mongolism coincided with great strides being made in medical genetics. The singular palmar crease identified by Reginald Langdon Down (son of John) hinted at chromosomal causes but the science of genetics had not progressed far enough for this to be verified or refuted. Despite invaluable contributions from mid- to late nineteenth-century scientists and medical practitioners, it was not until the early- to mid-twentieth century that important progress in medicine and genetics – with respect to mongolism – was made. At the International Congress of Genetics, Charles B. Davenport (1932) suggested that non-disjunction, an error in cell division in which an embryo has three copies of a chromosome instead of the usual two, was a cause of mongolism. A year later, UK geneticist and psychiatrist Lionel S. Penrose (1933) identified a partial correlation between mongolism and maternal age.

The work of Penrose, in particular, demonstrated how the connection between mental disability and hereditary factors was exaggerated. During this period, the vestiges of eugenic ideologies fostered the belief that intellectual disability was passed down hereditarily and was linked to social vices such as vagrancy, crime, and prostitution. These alleged connections hardened political attitudes to the unrestricted fertility of those defined as feeble-minded (Wright 2011). However, the many genetic investigations during this period mostly ended racial conjectures and marked the beginning of a genetic future. Penrose's claim that mongolism was associated with maternal age formed the basis of his 1949 landmark treatise *The Biology of Mental Defect*. In the same year, Barr and colleagues discovered that cells of male and female mammals could be distinguished by the presence or absence of a small, cellular body known as the sex chromatin. Present in females and absent in males, it could be used to determine sex in both humans and animals when sex chromosomes were unclear under the microscope.

One year later, in 1950, medical specialists and geneticists became interested in ascertaining foetal sex in cases of sex-related conditions such as haemophilia.[4] This was possible by using a new technology called amniocentesis, a diagnostic test carried out during pregnancy to assess the health of a foetus. Haemophilia diagnoses, at this time, were little more than tentative probability statements, but the discovery of Barr and his colleagues – and the use of amniocentesis – held promise for geneticists to be able to predict with greater certainty whether a foetus had the disorder (Macintyre 1973). In 1955, several different researchers in the USA, Denmark, and Israel were credited with discovering that the sex of foetuses could be predicted through analysing cells in the amniotic fluid (Cowan 1994).

Four years later, Dr Jérôme Lejeune (1959), a French physician and disability advocate, and colleagues made a ground-breaking discovery: mongolism was a chromosomal abnormality caused by the presence of three copies of chromosome 21, i.e. people with mongolism had forty-seven rather than forty-six chromosomes. In the same year, researchers also identified the link between chromosomes and both Turner syndrome[5] and Klinefelter syndrome[6] (Löwy 2014b). Researchers in the early 1960s (Clarke et al. 1961; Polani et al. 1960) also identified two rarer types of Down's syndrome, excepting the common form that was discovered by Lejeune and colleagues: Translocation Trisomy 21 and

Mosaic Trisomy 21 (both conditions are discussed in more detail later in this chapter). Lejeune and colleagues' discovery, giving rise to the name 'Trisomy 21' rather than mongolism or idiocy, was important in 'dramatising the medical value of human genetics', since doctors learned that many disorders had a genetic/chromosomal origin (Kevles 1995: 254). Although the culturing of foetal cells after an amniocentesis was initially difficult, this was resolved in 1966. In the same year, Lionel S. Penrose and George Smith published *Down's Anomaly*, widely considered to be the first medical textbook on the condition.

Giving birth to Down's syndrome and amniocentesis

Prenatal diagnostic techniques, allowing physicians to see 'what is about to be born' (Löwy 2014a: 154), have been developed in industrialised countries since the 1960s (Vassy 2005). The capacity to test in utero for chromosomal conditions, according to Kevles (1995) and Rapp (2000), legitimised amniocentesis and conferred on it the necessary value for scientific recognition as an integral tool for genetic diagnosis. In 1960, the first amniocentesis was used in Copenhagen to determine the sex of a foetus and subsequently offer a termination of pregnancy since the mother was identified as a carrier of haemophilia (Cowan 1994). It was at this point, then, that amniocentesis was recognised as a possible mechanism for prenatal diagnosis. It remained in its developmental stages for about fifteen years, because the safety and effectiveness of such techniques needed to be improved and because Scandinavia – where the first amniocentesis was used to terminate a pregnancy – was the only place, for much of that time, where 'eugenic therapeutic abortions' could be legally accessed (Cowan 1994: 38). Nonetheless, the development of amniocentesis paved the way for a rapid growth of medical genetics, meaning that prenatal diagnosis became strongly associated with genetic testing (Löwy 2014a).

In conjunction with the development of amniocentesis, the Abortion Act was implemented in the UK in 1967[7] and abortion laws were also liberalised in several Western democracies in the 1960s and 1970s (Löwy 2014a; Rapp 2000). Under section 1(1)(d) of the Abortion Act 1967, a pregnancy could be terminated 'up to term' where there was a risk that the child, if born, may be severely disabled and endanger the mental and physical health of the mother. The Human Fertilisation and Embryology Act 1990 amended the 1967 Abortion Act by creating a general upper limit of twenty-four weeks for termination except in circumstances where there was a serious risk to the pregnant woman's life or health, or there was a substantial risk of 'serious foetal abnormality'. Terminating a foetus that would 'suffer from physical or mental abnormalities as to be seriously handicapped', using the discourse of the 1967 Act, is still legal grounds for a termination of pregnancy in the UK, although what constitutes a 'serious handicap' is open to debate. In the same time period, an eminent group of biomedical researchers signed a letter objecting to the 'embarrassing term' of mongolism and proposed the substitution of this term with Trisomy 21, Langdon Down Anomaly, Down's Syndrome, Down's Anomaly, or Congenital Acromicria (Allen et al. 1961: 426). Similarly, in 1965, a Mongolian delegation approached the World Health Organisation (WHO) requesting that they, as well as others, stop using the term 'mongolism'. Whilst this change was accepted and implemented, it was still evident in scientific literature during the 1970s and has been used in recent leading medical texts (e.g. Underwood 2004). Nonetheless, it is at this point, officially at least, where one could claim that 'Down's syndrome' was born.

Deinstitutionalisation and community care

The birth of Down's syndrome and the onset of genetic testing coincided not only with abortion laws but, also, with the continued institutionalisation of people with the condition (Nancollas 2012). Prior to the 1970 Education Act, people with Down's syndrome mostly lived in state institutions (or asylums) and, according to Buckley and Buckley (2008), healthcare professionals still encouraged institutionalising children with the condition between the 1920s and 1960s. Despite such institutions being nationalised and transformed after the NHS was founded in 1948, persistent experimental treatments, sterilisations, lobotomies, and various forms of abuse were reported. Institutions were originally designed for moral treatment but they were crowded, non-therapeutic, lacked extensive funding, and isolated in location (Wright 2011). The moral therapy promised by institutions was supplanted by the custodial treatment of those inside the premises. Their mission moved from curing to maintaining, therapeutic considerations receding into the background as institutions became dumping grounds for 'social undesirables'; the 'once-grand asylums deteriorated into snake pits and hellholes worthy of exposés', warehouses for the discarded that isolated them physically and symbolically from the larger society (Geller and Morrissey 2004: 1128).

Over the course of the 1960s, people with disabilities – Down's syndrome included – were liberated from asylums in a process known as 'deinstitutionalisation', essentially 'a policy designed to reorganise mental health resources away from the institutions and into the community' (Wilson 1999: 252). The motives for deinstitutionalisation are multiple and contested, but Durham (1989) offers three reasons: a humanitarian concern for people with disabilities; the emergence of drug therapies; and economic factors (institutions were expensive to maintain). Arguably, deinstitutionalisation was also influenced by political denunciations and public backlashes against abuse, growing anti-psychiatry and pro-disability movements, evidence of the cognitive improvement of disabled people with access to a steady caregiver and consistent stimulation, and the rise of the popular premise that communities hold the capacity to de-stigmatise and advance the lives of those previously detained (Barton 1966; Goffman 1961; Stedman and Eichorn 1964; Szasz 1961). In the UK alone, the number of people living in institutions dropped from 154,000 in 1954 to 100,000 in 1982 (Pilgrim and Rogers 1993), although others argue that numbers dropped from 51,000 in 1976 to less than 4,000 in 2002 (Emerson 2004).

By the 1980s, people with conditions such as Down's syndrome were moved into the community under policies of inclusion and community provision that were supported by leading professionals in the fields of medicine and education (Nancollas 2012). The dominant strategy of community care at this time entailed the creation of group homes and making sure that clusters of adults with developmental disabilities lived in community settings. However, this policy was heavily criticised for many reasons including costs, the capacity of such sites to become mini-institutions, the difficulty of supervision that threatened residents' safety, and ambivalence among the general populace about having such places in *their* neighbourhoods. Yet, whilst the therapeutic intentions of deinstitutionalisation were not being met, the roots of this movement took shape and people were moved out of institutions. Since then, deinstitutionalisation has been critiqued due to minimal financial investment in alternative community-based treatment programmes, the purported abandonment of individuals with disabilities, the neglect of those unable to access adequate housing and other services, and its contribution to further stigmatising those who would have previously lived in asylum settings.

Down's syndrome and diagnostic testing

The inception of deinstitutionalisation overlapped with further developments in prenatal genetic testing. In 1968, Down's syndrome was detected via amniocentesis for the first time, but the use of this diagnostic technology was still sporadic owing to its 'experimental' status (Nadler 1968). In the same year and some time thereafter, researchers in Denmark (Mohr 1968; Hahnemann 1974) experimented with chorionic villus sampling (CVS) to identify genetic conditions – Down's syndrome included – in the first trimester of a pregnancy. Like amniocentesis, CVS is a prenatal diagnostic test carried out in pregnancy to assess foetal health. Widespread diagnostic testing via CVS and amniocentesis was adjourned at this stage but scientific research on Down's syndrome continued. In 1974, the condition was identified as possibly pathogenetic[8] (Neibuhr 1974) and the first mouse model[9] of Down's syndrome, Ts16, was created (Gropp et al. 1974). Gropp et al. (1975) created a new systematic model for studying chromosomal trisomies (such as Down's syndrome) in mice one year later. However, in 1980, it was discovered that this proposed mouse model failed as mice frequently died at, or near, birth (Polani and Adinolfi 1980).

Eight years after Down's syndrome was first detected using amniocentesis in 1968, the procedure became commonly used in the USA – helped by the introduction of public funds to finance it (Löwy 2014a) – and the first abortions following mid-trimester tests were reported (Global Down Syndrome Foundation 2012). For Cowan (1994), it was in 1975 and 1976 that amniocentesis extended beyond the 'developmental' stage and into the 'diffusion' stage. Rapp (2000: 33) identifies how the widespread use of prenatal diagnosis 'only became conceivable and possible when enrolled by and through legal access to abortion'. Since laws were reformed and therapeutic abortion, following the introduction of the Abortion Act 1967, had become legal in the UK (and other countries), the diffusion of amniocentesis was widespread. With it established as an acceptable part of reproductive practice, larger numbers of potential patients were anticipated after a presenting symptom of 'advanced maternal age', identified years earlier by Lionel S. Penrose, was recognised as more extensively distributed in the population compared to the previous indicator of a family history of sex-linked hereditary conditions (Cowan 1994). Offering diagnostic testing to mothers-to-be at an advanced maternal age was, therefore, seen as advisable.

Notably, the widespread uptake of amniocentesis was implicated in a number of legal cases during the late 1970s. During this period, there were instances in the USA where parents took legal action against hospitals for malpractice because the respective mother – aged over thirty-five – was not referred for amniocentesis and had a child with Down's syndrome. According to Löwy (2014b), the threat of litigation ignited a fear among professionals who wanted to both reduce the number of children born with an impairment (since they were viewed as a public health problem) and avoid legal action by expanding the scope of testing as well as the jurisdiction of the medical profession. Thus, it was the professionals' push, rather than the users' pull, that helped expand testing (Vassy 2005). In 1983, the American Congress of Obstetrics and Gynecologists and the American Academy of Pediatrics advised members that women over thirty-five years old should be mandatorily offered prenatal testing for genetic conditions including Down's syndrome. Additionally, Hook et al. (1983) published a paper suggesting that at a maternal age of thirty-five, the risk of having a baby with a chromosomal problem and the risk of having a miscarriage from an amniocentesis were both around 1 in 200. As such, the age of thirty-five was designated as the 'cut-off' for diagnostic testing, that is, of offering an amniocentesis to mothers-to-be aged thirty-five and above. This was because the risk of discovering a condition (0.5%) allegedly matched that of causing a miscarriage. Amniocentesis was subsequently offered exclusively to mothers-to-be aged thirty-five or above as opposed to *all* pregnant women (Wald et al. 1988).

It was not until the early- to mid-1990s that CVS came into common use (Cowan 1994). The trials of the technique in the late 1960s and early 1970s were largely unsuccessful and only in the early 1980s was CVS recognised as a possibly effective procedure for prenatal diagnosis, with a flurry of researchers using CVS to diagnose sex or chromosomal conditions and obtain tissue without causing a miscarriage (Cowan 1994). However, the development of CVS stalled for many years owing to the technique being difficult for professionals to learn (meaning that amniocentesis was preferred) and the obstruction of research with prohibitions against the use of federal funds, in light of the anti-abortion politics of the 1980s, to finance research in this area (Cowan 1994). In recent years, the technology has been improved and is currently used in UK obstetric practice.

Prenatal screening for Down's syndrome

Whilst diagnostic testing for Down's syndrome was developed and diffused from the late 1950s and early 1960s onwards, prenatal screening for the condition entered medical and scientific worlds in the latter stages of the twentieth century (as a reminder, prenatal *screening* precedes *diagnostic* testing and is used to identify women in whom a risk factor is deemed high enough to warrant offering diagnostic testing – more on this later in the chapter). Screening was largely introduced as an extension of earlier screening programmes for neural tube defects.[10] As one of the first instances of mass population screening used to detect a genetic condition, Down's syndrome screening began in the late 1980s following the discovery that low levels of alpha-fetoprotein (AFP)[11] in the mother's blood is associated with the condition (Cuckle et al. 1984) and the publication of Wald et al. (1988) on the possibility of carrying out 'maternal serum screening' for Down's syndrome. From this point onwards, Down's syndrome screening was introduced as a clinical service, with research carried out on data collected by patients after a screening procedure (Reynolds 2010). As such, research was frequently implemented without approval from research ethics committees and with no real governmental statement on the issue of screening for Down's syndrome. Nonetheless, the first routine screening programme for the condition in the NHS began in February 1990 in Newport and Cardiff (Wales, UK) during a one-year trial that was reported on three years later (Reynolds 2000). It purportedly took just two years of research to indicate the effectiveness of serum screening before it was made available to all mothers-to-be.

By 1998, many health authorities in the UK offered screening for Down's syndrome via serum screening for all parents-to-be regardless of age, although some offered age-restricted screening, that is, for mothers-to-be aged thirty-five and above only (Reynolds 2000). Most authorities offering screening used a 'double screen' which, rather than relying on maternal age or a history of a previously afflicted foetus and/or born child (Shaw et al. 2008), involved measuring two biochemical markers in the second trimester of pregnancy: alpha-fetoprotein (AFP) and total or free-beta human chorionic gonadotrophin (hCG).[12] Irrespective of the screening method used, parents-to-be were categorised as 'screen-positive' (higher-risk) or 'screen-negative' (lower-risk) which was used to guide decisions around diagnostic testing. The performance of the screening was established by measuring a detection rate and false-positive rate. The false-positive rate was crucial as it indicated the number of unaffected pregnancies subjected to diagnostic tests that could cause problems, such as miscarriage (Harrison and Goldie 2006).[13] However, due to the low detection rate and poor cost-effectiveness of the double screen (Shaw et al. 2008), the 'triple screen' was developed. The triple screen, first described in the UK in 1988 (Canick et al. 1988) but implemented years later, improved the double screen by measuring ue3 (unconjugated estriol),[14] with AFP and hCG, and offered an improved detection rate and reduced false-positive rate (Wald et al. 1988).

Around this time, the search for serum markers for a 'risk' of Down's syndrome was combined with another approach to detect such a risk: obstetrical ultrasound (Löwy 2014b). Ultrasound was introduced to the investigation of pregnancy in the late 1950s to diagnose hydramnios, hydatidiform mole,[15] twin pregnancy, and pregnancies with a high risk of miscarriage. Over the years, the relationship between ultrasound and biochemical tests intensified the routine use of ultrasound and helped transform it into an independent prenatal tool. This routinisation was influenced, also, by the visualisation of the foetus (via ultrasound) and developments in medical photography (e.g. Lennart Nilsson's pictures of developing embryos published in *Life* magazine in 1965) that ensured the 'foetal patient' became an object of both public and academic discussion (Mitchell 2001).

Although the double screen for Down's syndrome was initially favoured over the triple screen (Reynolds 2010), the triple screen became the most commonly used technique for Down's syndrome screening in the UK between 2000 and 2010 (NHS FASP 2012). This emerged despite the development of the 'quadruple screen' which involves measuring the same biochemical markers as a triple screen, plus inhibin-A,[16] around fifteen to eighteen weeks into a pregnancy. This was reported to have an improved detection rate and false-positive rate in comparison with the triple screen (Malone et al. 2005). In 2006, the UK National Screening Committee (NSC) – implementing a national screening policy – recommended using quadruple screening for achieving a 75% detection rate and 3% false-positive rate for Down's syndrome (Harrison and Goldie 2006; Wald et al. 2003). Quadruple screening did not initially surpass triple screening on account of various complications that affected the capacity to produce an accurate result in the laboratory. The reluctance to fully embrace quadruple screening in the UK, for Reynolds (2010), could also be attributed to diminishing returns in relation to economic cost, an incremental improvement of detection being less with each extra analyte[17] added, and the wishes of parents-to-be to undertake an earlier test (in the first trimester). But in more recent years, its complications have been resolved and quadruple screening has subsequently been used ahead of triple screening in clinical practice (Harrison and Goldie 2006). Indeed, triple screening has not been offered anywhere in the UK since 2012 (NHS FASP 2012).

Despite improvements in screening for Down's syndrome (performed in the second trimester), there were calls for first trimester screening to be offered in the UK, primarily because it was predicted that it could help fulfil the NSC's desire to develop a screening programme offering a 75% detection rate and 3% false-positive rate. The initial development of first trimester screening for Down's syndrome followed research by Nicolaides et al. (1992) and Snijders et al. (1998) who suggested that a nuchal translucency measurement (the fluid thickness in the nape of a foetal neck) obtained via an ultrasound scan could be used as a possible marker for Down's syndrome and other genetic conditions. The first screening programme developed for the first trimester of pregnancy was 'combined screening'. This involved combining the results from an ultrasound scan and biochemical serum screening – hCG and pregnancy associated plasma protein A (PAPP-A)[18] – at around eleven to fourteen weeks gestation. The association between Down's syndrome and low levels of PAPP-A and high levels of hCG during the first trimester was first reported during the early 1990s (Wald et al. 1992). The ultrasound scan involved measuring both the crown rump length (CRL)[19] and nuchal translucency of a foetus. Combined screening offered improved detection and false-positive rates in comparison to all methods of second trimester screening (Malone et al. 2005) and quickened the process of receiving concrete results as CVS could be carried out in the first trimester whilst amniocentesis could not (Shaw et al. 2008).

In the 2000s, other screening methods were developed (serum integrated screening, integrated screening, contingent screening) but these were not widely used in the UK (Shaw et al. 2008). Despite often promising higher detection rates and lower false-positive rates, such techniques were overlooked since they were costly, they could delay results because they required collecting data in both trimesters, they required parents-to-be to attend the clinic on at least two occasions (risking dropouts), and they could involve withholding information about a first-trimester result, a move which could be viewed as unethical practice (Reynolds 2010). At the time of writing, Down's syndrome screening standards imposed by the NHS Foetal Anomaly Screening Programme (NHS FASP 2012), a UK organisation dedicated to ensuring access to a uniform screening programme, claims that screening should be done using the combined screen, serum integrated screen, or integrated screen in the first trimester or the quadruple screen in the second semester (Reynolds 2010). An annual report produced by NHS FASP (2012) suggests that, in 2011 and 2012, the main screening method offered by hospitals in England alone was combined screening (86% and 96% respectively), with those parents-to-be who book too late for combined screening (first trimester) alternatively being offered a quadruple screen (second trimester).

Down's syndrome screening and testing: Freymarsh and Springtown

So far in this chapter, I have outlined a concise socio-history of Down's syndrome and screening/testing for the condition. The remainder of the chapter describes the background and possible symptoms of Down's syndrome and outlines current screening and testing practices in the two research sites: Freymarsh and Springtown. This also includes a short explanation about how maternal age is implicated in an increased chance of a foetus being diagnosed with the condition. This provides the necessary context of my study and draws attention to current practices that establish Down's syndrome as a site worthy of critical attention.

Down's syndrome: the condition

The human body is made up of cells containing genes which are enclosed within thread-like structures. These are referred to as chromosomes, that is, the packages of genetic material or deoxyribonucleic acid (DNA) stored within the nucleus of each cell. They contain instructions for how the body's cells develop together with the eye colour and sex of a foetus. A human usually has forty-six chromosomes organised into twenty-three pairs (twenty-two autosomal pairs and one pair of sex chromosomes) inherited from the mother-to-be and father-to-be. Genetic diversity among different people is generated via the exchange of genetic material between chromosomes (meiosis I) and the separation of chromosome pairs (meiosis II). When an egg is fertilised to create a new cell (zygote), new pairs of chromosomes are created in which each parent-to-be contributes one chromosome to each pair. On occasions, an error occurs in which there is a failure of the chromosomal pairs to separate (non-disjunction). This causes an imbalance of chromosomes ('aneuploidy'). A cell *losing* a chromosome ('monosomy') is likely to be lethal, but this is not always the case when a cell *gains* a chromosome ('trisomy'), causing three copies of a chromosome instead of a usual pair.

One form of trisomy (when there are more than forty-six chromosomes) is Down's syndrome (or Trisomy 21), caused by the presence of an extra chromosome on the twenty-first pairing. The condition is the most common trisomy that is detected during pregnancy, followed by Edward's syndrome and Patau syndrome. Down's syndrome is an incurable chromosomal condition which occurs in one to two of every 1,000 live births in the UK (NHS 2015). It is one of the most common genetic causes of learning disability and most people with the condition (94% of all cases) have Full Trisomy 21 Down's syndrome, whilst 4% of cases have Translocation Down's syndrome and 2% of cases have Mosaic Down's syndrome. Children with Translocation Down's syndrome have extra chromosome 21 material attached to another chromosome. Only Translocation Down's syndrome can be hereditary. Some people do not have symptoms of Translocation Down's syndrome but they can be a carrier, meaning that they have altered genes that trigger the condition in their unborn children. The risk of 'passing on' the condition depends on the sex of the carrier, with mothers-to-be more likely to 'pass' the condition onto a child. Mosaic Down's syndrome is caused by the mis-division of chromosomes *after* fertilisation during early cell division. Whilst children with Full Trisomy 21 have an extra copy of chromosome 21 in every cell, children with Mosaic Trisomy 21 have an extra chromosome 21 in only some cells.

Whilst symptoms of the condition vary between each case, common symptoms of Down's syndrome include an upward eye slant, large tongue, clinodactyly,[20] single transverse palm crease,[21] sandal gap,[22] excess skin on the back of the neck, a flat facial profile, brushfield spots,[23] weak muscle tone, and umbilical hernia (CARIS 2012). People with the condition may also have impaired cognitive abilities, a reduced IQ, learning difficulties, and restricted physical growth. They may also be more susceptible to ear infections, bronchitis, colds, and pneumonia than people without the condition. Females with Down's syndrome can have fertility problems and males with the condition are often infertile (CARIS 2012). The outlook of life for a person with Down's syndrome can vary widely. This depends on whether a child develops serious health conditions, such as sight and hearing loss, intestinal problems, hearing and vision problems, thyroid complications, dementia, Alzheimer's disease, and leukaemia (NHS 2015). Around 50% of children with Down's syndrome have a congenital heart defect and around 60% of this group require treatment in hospital. By contrast, the condition seems to offer protection against some cancers and cardiovascular disease. Importantly, however, people with Down's syndrome can experience few or several of these complications (NHS 2015).

There is no medical 'cure' for the condition but Down's syndrome is frequently demarcated as 'not lethal' (Ivry 2009), meaning that individuals with the condition are likely to survive childbirth and can enjoy a good 'quality of life' (Buckley and Buckley 2008; CARIS 2012; NHS FASP 2012). On the NHS website (NHS 2015), it is claimed that there are many ways in which children with the condition can develop into 'healthy and fulfilled individuals' who can enjoy access to healthcare and early intervention programmes and possibly achieve independence. Similarly, Buckley and Buckley (2008) suggest that support for people with the condition is better than the past and their current medical needs are largely understood; several healthcare professionals, for instance, may monitor/treat people with Down's syndrome, including physiotherapists, speech and language therapists, ophthalmologists, occupational therapists, audiologists, dieticians, general practitioners, paediatricians, and cardiologists (NHS 2015). Adults with Down's syndrome can pursue further education, gain employment, and live independently (Buckley and Buckley 2008). Additionally, according to Buckley and Buckley (2008: 84), people with the condition are rarely anti-social or violent and, whilst they can experience challenges, they can 'make positive contributions to family and community life and often form loving and caring relationships'.

However, whilst the progress of people with the condition has been remarkable in the past fifty years, the prognosis of the condition is still uncertain. It is extremely difficult, if not impossible, to predict how a child will be affected in the future. Nonetheless, due to medical advances and better knowledge of treatment and care options, children born with Down's syndrome – most of which are diagnosed postnatally – are today likely to survive beyond sixty years (CARIS 2012). This has significantly increased from nine years old in 1929, twelve years old in 1946, twenty-five years old in 1983, and forty-nine years old in 1997 (Penrose 1949; Yang et al. 2002).

The object of screening at Freymarsh and Springtown

In the UK, all parents-to-be are offered prenatal screening for Down's syndrome, which cannot establish a diagnosis but can assist reproductive decision-making regarding diagnostic testing. Screening should take place in a window of ten to twenty weeks during a pregnancy, although the preferred period of time is by the end of the first trimester (thirteen weeks and six days gestation). During my fieldwork at two clinics – Freymarsh (NHS hospital) and Springtown (privately funded clinic) – two screening methods were used: quadruple screening (Freymarsh) and combined screening (Springtown). The quadruple screen can detect approximately 75% of affected pregnancies with a 3% false-positive rate. In contrast, combined screening can detect around 85% of affected pregnancies with a lower false-positive rate (CARIS 2012). Irrespective of the screening method, parents-to-be receive a 'risk factor', a numeric ratio establishing the odds of a foetus having Down's syndrome. The screening methods at Freymarsh and Springtown are based on the same mathematical principle and work by combining a prior probability – maternal age at expected date of delivery – with a likelihood ratio based on several factors such as weight, gestation, ethnicity, pregnancy history, smoking habits, the number of foetuses, and whether it is an assisted conception. At Springtown, these factors are combined with the size of a nuchal translucency detected via ultrasound.[24] Taken together, these create an estimate of whether a foetus has Down's syndrome.

Three risk factors are produced at Freymarsh: a background risk (based on age, ethnicity, previous history, etc.), a biochemistry risk (based on measurements of four biochemical markers detected via screening), and an adjusted risk (based on combining a background risk and biochemistry risk). At Springtown, these same three risk factors are produced alongside an ultrasound risk (based on the nuchal translucency size alone). In Freymarsh and Springtown, only the adjusted risk factor is referred to when delivering a result to parents-to-be. In addition, whilst only a risk factor for Down's syndrome is given to parents-to-be in Freymarsh, parents-to-be in Springtown also receive risk factors for Edward's syndrome and Patau syndrome. This reflects a shift in modern biomedical practice from the actual to the potential, redefining the idea of 'the patient' to include those 'at-risk'.

In Freymarsh and Springtown, the cut-off point for categorising a pregnancy as 'at-risk', or not, is 1:150 (a 1 in 150 risk of having a foetus with Down's syndrome).[25] If parents-to-be receive a risk factor numerically higher than 1:150 (e.g. 1:250), they are categorised as 'lower-risk' and receive a letter notifying them of this (at Springtown, they receive a telephone call). At this point, parents-to-be are not offered or advised to have further treatment except for an ultrasound at twenty weeks to check for other potential issues ('anomaly scan'). In contrast, if parents-to-be receive a risk factor numerically lower than 1:150 (e.g. 1:100), they are categorised as 'higher-risk' and diagnostic testing (i.e. amniocentesis or CVS) is offered to prove or refute a suspected diagnosis. Around 3–5% of pregnant women in England and Wales who consent to screening receive a higher-risk result (NHS FASP 2012), and according to Buckley and Buckley (2008), between one in twenty and one in thirty higher-risk (screen-positive) results lead to a diagnosis of Down's syndrome.[26]

The object of testing at Freymarsh and Springtown

Diagnostic testing for Down's syndrome involves undertaking an amniocentesis or CVS. An amniocentesis involves taking a small sample of amniotic fluid by passing a fine needle through the abdomen of a mother-to-be and drawing the fluid out using a syringe. During CVS, a small sample of placenta is taken either by passing a small needle through the abdomen of a mother-to-be and drawing the fluid out using a syringe, or by passing a small tube through a vagina and cervix. CVS is carried out in the first trimester after ten weeks of a pregnancy and an amniocentesis is often carried out in the second trimester between fifteen and twenty weeks gestation. Amniocentesis can also be carried out late in a pregnancy to check foetal well-being and to potentially diagnose a condition (but not for the purpose of termination). Amniocentesis and CVS provide an accurate diagnosis but have a few possible complications such as causing miscarriage, infection, bleeding, and premature labour. The risk of miscarriage is reported as being 1% due to amniocentesis and 2% due to CVS (Buckley and Buckley 2008).

Diagnostic testing is offered because of a possible indication of a genetic condition, previous or current pregnancy complications, a family history of a condition, and an advanced maternal age (although this last option is currently not common in UK medicine). After diagnostic testing is completed, samples are sent to a cytogenetic laboratory. Cytogenetics is concerned with the function and structure of cells, especially chromosomes. Two results are possible after testing in the cytogenetics laboratory: a QF-PCR (quantitative fluorescence polymerase chain reaction) result and a full karyotype. A QF-PCR result includes an amplification, detection, and analysis of chromosome-specific DNA sequences. This provides a conclusive diagnosis for Down's syndrome, Edward's syndrome, Patau syndrome, and sex chromosome aneuploidies such as Turner syndrome and Klinefelter syndrome. Since QF-PCR misses some chromosomal conditions, it is followed by a full karyotype. This involves analysing all chromosomes in detail at the microscopic level for chromosome deletions, duplications, translocations, inversions, and insertions. Such methods reveal chromosomal conditions other than those specified above, together with any abnormal genes. Although a QF-PCR result is usually available in less than two days following a procedure, a full karyotype is available approximately two weeks after this period in both Freymarsh and Springtown. After a result is established, this information is returned to professionals who must deliver this news to parents-to-be. If a diagnosis is established, counselling is offered before a decision has to be made about whether to continue or terminate a pregnancy. The main objective of screening is to identify women in whom a risk factor is deemed high enough to warrant offering them diagnostic testing.

Maternal age and Down's syndrome

Whilst it is not fully understood why some babies are conceived with abnormal copies of chromosomes, maternal age is the only clear factor which is known to increase the chance of having a baby with Down's syndrome (NHS 2015). The reason for this relationship remains unclear, but what is observable is that, despite higher pregnancy rates among mothers under thirty-five years old (ONS 2011), more babies with the condition are born to mothers aged thirty-five and above (CARIS 2012). According to a handbook that is published for professionals at Freymarsh, a mother-to-be who is sixteen years old has a maternal age risk, prior to any form of screening, of 1:1509 (i.e. a 1 in 1509 chance that a foetus has Down's syndrome). This increases to 1:1476 at the age of twenty, 1:1339 at twenty-five, and 1:937 at thirty. At the age of thirty-five, a maternal age risk is 1:352. This increases to 1:266 at thirty-six, 1:199 at thirty-seven, 1:148 at thirty-eight, 1:111 at thirty-nine, and 1:85 at forty. At the age of forty-five, the maternal age risk for Down's syndrome is 1:35. A report conducted by the NDSCR (Morris and Springett 2014) claims that in 2013 in England and Wales, 102 women aged twenty-four and below had a prenatal or postnatal diagnosis of Down's syndrome (5% of all diagnoses). This compared to 175 women aged twenty-five to twenty-nine (9% of all diagnoses), 327 women aged thirty to thirty-four (17% of all diagnoses), 603 women aged thirty-five to thirty-nine (32% of all diagnoses), 457 women aged forty to forty-four (24% of all diagnoses), and 42 women aged forty-five and above (2% of all diagnoses).[27]

Summary

In this chapter, I initially provided a short socio-history that captured how Down's syndrome has become a critical site in prenatal care and how it has been drawn into reproductive politics through entwining social, technological, scientific, legal, economic, political, and cultural developments. By studying the condition and its intersection with prenatal care historically, I unmasked the practices and values that we now take for granted and highlighted how the transformation of prenatal diagnosis into a routine medical technology represents what Löwy (2014b: 296) calls an 'invisible revolution, hidden in plain sight'. The likes of Lejeune and Penrose were unlikely to be aware, in the first instance, of the potential their findings had for detecting and terminating foetuses with Down's syndrome. However, this is the situation that prenatal medicine now finds itself in. In what followed, I described Down's syndrome, its possible symptoms, how it is screened and testing for at both Freymarsh and Springtown, and how maternal age is associated with the condition. This chapter, in its entirety, provides the necessary context for the next four chapters in which I present data from my study.

Notes

1 For related historical accounts of disability and the evolution of ideas around disablement, see: Carlson (2009); Danforth (2009); Longmore and Umansky (2001), and; Stiker (2000).

2 I am aware that the terms mongolism and idiocy are likely to cause offence to UK and international advocacy organisations as well as parents of children with the condition. This is not my intention and I argue that their use here is integral to fully detail the history and making of Down's syndrome. I return to the importance of disability-related discourse later in the book. Hereafter, I will not use quotation marks around historical terms.

3 Although the diagnostic category of Down's syndrome was first described in the nineteenth century, Starbuck (2011) identifies skeletal remains and different forms of material culture (paintings, figurines, pottery) that may depict Down's syndrome well before this period. Another example of an artistic representation is the painting *The Adoration of the Christ Child* that includes an angelic figure whose facial features appear to represent a person with Down's syndrome (Levinas and Reid 2003).

4 Haemophilia is an inherited genetic disorder that impairs the ability to form blood clots.

5 Turner syndrome is a genetic disorder which only affects females. A female with the condition will have all or part of one X chromosome missing.

6 Klinefelter syndrome is the set of symptoms resulting from extra X genetic material in males. Symptoms may not be obvious and can vary significantly among individuals.

7 For reflections on the possible reasons for the changing public views of abortion in the global North – including feminist struggles, greater sexual freedom, women's increased participation in the workforce, the wider publicity of abortion, the thalidomide scandal of 1961–1962 and the rubella epidemics of 1962–1965, and concerns about unequal access to safe abortions – see: Löwy (2014b).

8 Pathogenic is a medical term describing viruses, bacteria, and other germs that can cause disease.

9 A mouse model is a strain of mice used in scientific research to study a condition or disease that occurs in human populations. Animal models are used to determine whether specific treatment options are effective and if they could be used on humans.

10 Neural tube defects are birth defects of the brain, spine, or spinal cord. The two most common neural tube defects are spina bifida and anencephaly.

11 Alpha-fetoprotein (AFP) is a protein in humans encoded by the AFP gene produced during foetal development.

12 Total or free-beta human chorionic gonadotrophin (hCG) is a hormone produced after pregnancy conception.
13 The selection of a cut-off is decided by a choice between affected live births prevented and unaffected foetuses lost (Buckley and Buckley 2008).
14 Estriol is one of the main three oestrogens produced by the human body.
15 A hydatidiform mole (or molar pregnancy) is a growing mass of tissue inside a womb that will not develop into a foetus.
16 Inhibin-A is a hormone that is produced by the placenta during a pregnancy.
17 An analyte is a substance or chemical constituent that is the subject of chemical analysis.
18 Pregnancy associated plasma protein A (PAPP-A) is the largest pregnancy associated protein produced by the embryo and placenta.
19 Crown rump length (CRL) is the measurement of the length of a foetus from the top of the head to the bottom of the buttocks.
20 Clinodactyly is the curvature of a finger or toe.
21 Single transverse palmar crease is a single crease that extends across the palm of the hand.
22 Sandal gap refers to an apparent increase in interspace between the first toe (great toe) and the second toe.
23 Brushfield spots are small spots on the periphery of the iris in the human eye.
24 Some clinics will also take account of the presence/absence of a nasal bone, another marker of Down's syndrome and other chromosomal conditions (Cicero et al. 2001). However, Springtown do not usually offer this service owing to a lack of training among the sonographers working there.
25 This varies between countries and depends on political and economic factors, along with whether national screening policies are established. According to Boyd et al. (2008), for example, diagnostic tests are routinely offered to mothers-to-be aged thirty-five and above in Germany and Spain independent of a risk factor.
26 Suspicions of Down's syndrome can also be established during an anomaly scan that is performed at twenty weeks gestation. The absence of a nasal bone, an increased nuchal translucency, cardiac defects, or an echogenic bowel (when the appearance of a foetal bowel on an ultrasound scan is brighter than usual) can indicate a potential diagnosis of the condition.
27 According to Morris and Springett (2014), 180 (10% of all cases) cases are missing.

Bibliography

Allen, G., Benda, C.E., Böök, J.A., Carter, C.O., Ford, C.E., Chu, E.H.Y., Hanhart, E., Jervis, G.A., Langdon Down, W., Lejeune, J., Nishimura, H., Oster, J., Penrose, L.S., Polani, P.E., Potter, E.L., Stern, C., Turpin, R., Warkany, J. and Yannet, H. 1961. Letter to the editor. *Lancet* 1(775), p. 426.
Barton, R. 1966. *Institutional Neurosis*. Bristol: Wright and Sons.
Bérubé, M. 1996. *Life As We Know It: A Father, a Family, and an Exceptional Child*. New York: Pantheon Books.
Boyd, P.A., DeVigan, C., Khoshnood, B., Loane, M., Garne, E., Dolk, H. and the EUROCAT Working Group. 2008. Survey of prenatal screening policies in Europe for structural malformations and chromosome anomalies, and their impact on detection and termination rates for neural tube defects and Down's syndrome. *BJOG: An International Journal of Obstetrics and Gynaecology* 115(6), pp. 689–696.

Buckley, F. and Buckley, S.J. 2008. Wrongful deaths and rightful lives: screening for Down syndrome. *Down Syndrome Research and Practice* 12(2), pp. 79–86.

Canick, J.A., Knight, G.J., Palomaki, G.E., Haddow, J.E., Cuckle, H.S. and Wald, N.J. 1988. Low second trimester maternal serum unconjugated oestriol in pregnancies with Down's syndrome. *British Journal of Obstetrics and Gynaecology* 95(4), pp. 330–333.

CARIS. 2012. *CARIS Review 2012*. Swansea: Public Health Wales.

Carlson, L. 2009. *The Faces of Intellectual Disability: Philosophical Reflections*. Bloomington: Indiana University Press.

Casper, M.J. and Clarke, A.E. 1998. Making the Pap smear into the 'right tool' for the job: cervical cancer screening in the USA, circa 1940–1995. *Social Studies of Science* 28(2), pp. 255–290.

Cicero, S., Curcio, P., Papageorghiou, A., Sonek, J. and Nicolaides, K. 2001. Absence of nasal bone in fetuses with trisomy 21 at 11–14 weeks of gestation: an observational study. *Lancet* 358(9294), pp. 1665–1667.

Clarke, C.M., Edwards, J.H. and Smallpiece, V. 1961. 21-trisomy/normal mosaicism in an intelligent child with some Mongoloid characters. *Lancet* 1(7185), pp. 1028–1030.

Cowan, R.S. 1994. Women's roles in the history of amniocentesis and chorionic villi sampling. In: Rothenberg, K. and Thomson, E. eds. *Women and Prenatal Testing: Facing the Challenges of Genetic Technology*. Columbus: Ohio State University Press, pp. 35–48.

Cuckle, H.S., Wald, N.J. and Lindenbaum, R.H. 1984. Maternal serum alpha-fetoprotein measurement: a screening test for Down syndrome. *Lancet* 323(8383), pp. 926–929.

Danforth, S. 2009. *The Incomplete Child: An Intellectual History of Learning Disabilities*. Oxford: Peter Lang.

Davenport, C.B. 1932. *International Congress of Genetics: Mendelism in Man* [Online]. Available at: www.esp.org/books/6th-congress/facsimile/contents/6th-cong-p135-davenport.pdf [Accessed: 7 August 2016].

Down, J.L.H. [1866] 1997. Observations on an ethnic classification of idiots [Online]. Available at: www.neonatology.org/classics/down.html [Accessed: 7 August 2016].

Durham, M.L. 1989. The impact of deinstitutionalization on the current treatment of the mentally ill. *International Journal of Law and Psychiatry* 12(2–3), pp. 117–131.

Emerson, E. 2004. Deinstitutionalisation in England. *Journal of Intellectual and Developmental Disability* 29(1), pp. 79–84.

Esquirol, J.E.D. 1838. *Des Maladies Mentales Considérées Sous les Rapports Médical, Hygiénique et Médico-légal, Volume 1*. Paris: J.B. Baillière.

Galton, F. 1883. *Inquiries into Human Faculty and Its Development*. London: Macmillan.

Geller, J.L. and Morrissey, J.P. 2004. Asylum within and without asylum. *Hospital and Community Psychiatry* 55(10), pp. 1128–1130.

Giddens, A. 1991. *Modernity and Self-Identity: Self and Society in the Late Modern Age*. Cambridge: Polity Press.

Global Down Syndrome Foundation. 2012. History of Down syndrome: medical care and research [Online]. Available at: www.globaldownsyndrome.org/about-down-syndrome/history-of-down-syndrome/?page_id=4578 [Accessed: 7 August 2016].

Goffman, E. 1961. *Asylums: Essays on the Social Situation of Mental Patients and Other Inmates*. Harmondsworth: Penguin Books.

Gropp, A., Giers, D. and Kolbus, U. 1974. Trisomy in the fetal backcross progeny of male and female metacentric heterozygotes of the mouse. *Cytogenetic and Genome Research* 13(6), pp. 511–535.

Gropp, A., Kolbus, U. and Giers, D. 1975. Systematic approach to the study of trisomy in the mouse. *Cytogenetic and Genome Research* 14(1), pp. 42–62.

Hahnemann, N. 1974. Early prenatal diagnosis: a study of biopsy techniques and cell culturing from extraembryonic membranes. *Clinical Genetics* 6(4), pp. 294–306.

Harrison, G. and Goldie, D. 2006. Second-semester Down's syndrome serum screening: double, triple, or quadruple marker testing? *Annals of Clinical Biochemistry* 43(1), pp. 67–72.

Hook, E.B., Cross, P.K. and Schreinemachers, D.M. 1983. Chromosomal abnormality rates at amniocentesis and in live-born infants. *Journal of American Medical Association* 249(15), pp. 2034–2038.

Ivry, T. 2009. The ultrasonic picture show and the politics of threatened life. *Medical Anthropology Quarterly* 23(3), pp. 189–211.

Kevles, D. 1995. *In the Name of Eugenics: Genetics and the Uses of Human Heredity.* Cambridge, MA: Harvard University Press.

Lejeune, J., Turpin, R. and Gautier, M. 1959. Le mongolisme. Premier exemple d'aberration autosomique humaine. *Annales de Génétique* 1(2), pp. 41–49.

Levinas, A.S. and Reid, C.S. 2003. An angel with Down syndrome in a sixteenth century Flemish nativity painting. *American Journal of Medical Genetics* 116A(4), pp. 399–405.

Lifton, R.J. 1986. *The Nazi Doctors: Medical Killing and the Psychology of Genocide.* New York: Basic Books.

Logan, J. 2011. A brief history of Down syndrome, part 1: how Down syndrome got its name (31 for 21 challenge, day 11). *Down With Dat.* Weblog [Online] 11 October. Available from: http://downwitdat.blogspot.ca/2013/07/a-brief-history-of-down-syndrome-part-1.html [Accessed: 7 August 2016].

Longmore, P.K. and Umansky, L. 2001. *The New Disability History: American Perspectives.* New York: New York University Press.

Löwy, I. 2014a. How genetics came to the unborn. *Studies in History of Philosophy of Biological and Biomedical Sciences* 47(Part A), pp. 154–162.

Löwy, I. 2014b. Prenatal diagnosis: the irresistible rise of the 'visible foetus'. *Studies in History of Philosophy of Biological and Biomedical Sciences* 47(Part B), pp. 290–299.

Macintyre, M.N. 1973. Genetic risk, prenatal diagnosis and selective abortion. In: Walbert, D.F. and Butler, D. eds. *Abortion, Society and the Law.* Cleveland, OH: Case Western Reserve University Press, pp. 234–252.

Malone, F.D., Canick, J.A., Ball, R.H., Nyberg, D.A., Comstock, C.H., Bukowski, R., Berkowitz, R.L., Gross, S.J., Dugoff, L., Craigo, S.D., Timor-Tritsch, I.E., Carr, S.R., Wolfe, H.M., Dukes, K., Bianchi, D.W., Rudnicka, A.R., Hackshaw, A.K., Lambert-Messerlian, G., Wald, N.J. and D'Alton, M.E. 2005. First-trimester or second-trimester screening, or both, for Down's syndrome. *New England Journal of Medicine* 353(19), pp. 2001–2011.

Mitchell, L.M. 2001. *Baby's First Picture: Ultrasound and the Politics of Fetal Subjects.* Toronto: University of Toronto Press.

Mohr, J. 1968. Foetal genetic diagnosis: development of techniques for early sampling of foetal cells. *Acta Pathologica et Microbiologica Scandinavia* 73(1), pp. 73–77.

Morris, J.K. and Springett, A. 2014. *The National Down Syndrome Cytogenetic Register for England and Wales: 2013 Annual Report.* London: Wolfson Institute of Preventive Medicine.

Nadler, H.L. 1968. Antenatal detection of hereditary disorders. *Paediatrics* 42(6), pp. 912–918.

Nancollas, C. 2012. *Down's Syndrome: The Biography*. London: Darton Longman and Todd.

Neibuhr, E. 1974. The possibility of a pathogenetic segment on chromosome 21. *Humangenetik* 21(1), pp. 99–101.

NHS. 2015. Down's syndrome. *NHS Choices* [Online]. Available at: www.nhs.uk/Conditions/Downs-syndrome/Pages/Introduction.aspx?url=Pages/what-is-it.aspx [Accessed: 7 August 2016].

NHS FASP. 2012. *NHS Fetal Anomaly Screening Programme: Annual Report 2011–2012*. University of Exeter: NHS Fetal Anomaly Screening Programme.

Nicolaides, K.H., Azar, G., Byrne, D., Mansur, C. and Marks, K. 1992. Fetal nuchal translucency: ultrasound screening for chromosomal defects in first trimester of pregnancy. *British Medical Journal* 304(6831), pp. 867–869.

ONS. 2011. *Statistical Bulletin: Live Births in England and Wales by Characteristics of Mother 1, 2011*. Newport: Office for National Statistics.

Penrose, L.S. 1933. The relative effect of paternal and maternal age in mongolism. *Journal of Genetics* 27(2), pp. 219–224.

Penrose, L.S. 1949. The incidence of mongolism in the general population. *British Journal of Psychiatry* 95(400), pp. 685–688.

Pilgrim, D. and Rogers, A. 1993. *A Sociology of Mental Health and Illness*. Buckingham: Open University Press.

Polani, P.E. and Adinolfi, M. 1980. Chromosome 21 of man, 22 of the great apes and 16 of the mouse. *Developmental Medicine and Child Neurology* 22(2), pp. 223–225.

Polani, P.E., Briggs, J.H., Ford, C.E., Clarke, C.M. and Berg, J.M. 1960. A mongol girl with 46 chromosomes. *Lancet* 1(7127), pp. 721–724.

Proctor, R.B. 1988. *Racial Hygiene: Medicine Under the Nazis*. Cambridge, MA: Harvard University Press.

Pueschel, S.M. 2000. *A Parent's Guide to Down Syndrome: Towards a Brighter Future*. New York: Brookes Publishing.

Rapp, R. 2000. *Testing Women, Testing the Fetus: The Social Impact of Amniocentesis in America*. London: Routledge.

Reynolds, T. 2000. Down's syndrome screening: a controversial test, with more controversy to come! *Journal of Clinical Pathology* 53(12), pp. 893–898.

Reynolds, T. 2010. The triple test as a screening technique for Down syndrome: reliability and relevance. *International Journal of Women's Health* 2, pp. 83–88.

Séguin, É. 1846. *Traitment Moral, Hygiène et Éducation des Idiots et des Autres Enfants Arriérés*. Paris: J.B. Baillière.

Selikowitz, M. 2008. *Down Syndrome: The Facts*. 3rd edn. Oxford: Oxford University Press.

Shaw, S.W., Hsu, J.J., Lee, C.N., Hsiao, C.H., Chen, C.P., Hsieh, T.T. and Cheng, P.J. 2008. First and second-trimester Down syndrome screening: current strategies and clinical guidelines. *Taiwan Journal of Obstetrics and Gynecology* 47(2), pp. 157–162.

Snijders, R.J., Noble, P., Sebire, N., Souka, A. and Nicolaides, K.H. 1998. UK multicentre project on assessment of risk of trisomy 21 by maternal age and fetal nuchal-translucency thickness at 10–14 weeks of gestation. *Lancet* 352(9125), pp. 343–346.

Starbuck, J.M. 2011. On the antiquity of Trisomy 21: moving towards a quantitative diagnosis of Down syndrome in historic material culture. *Journal of Contemporary Anthropology* 2(1), pp. 62–89.

Stedman, D.J. and Eichorn, D.H. 1964. A comparison of the growth and development of institutionalized and home-reared mongoloids during infancy and early childhood. *American Journal of Mental Deficiency* 69(3), 391–401.

Stiker, H.J. 2000. *A History of Disability*. Ann Arbor: University of Michigan Press.

Szasz, T.S. 1961. *The Myth of Mental Illness: Foundations of a Theory of Personal Conduct*. London: Secker and Warburg.

Underwood, J.C.E. 2004. *General and Systematic Pathology*. 4th edn. London: Churchill Livingstone.

Vassy, C. 2005. How prenatal diagnosis became acceptable in France. *Trends in Biotechnology* 23(5), pp. 246–249.

Wald, N.J., Cuckle, H.S., Densem, J.W., Nanchalal, K., Royston, P., Chard, T., Haddow, J.E., Knight, G.J., Palomaki, G.E. and Canick, J.A. 1988. Maternal serum screening for Down's syndrome in early pregnancy. *British Medical Journal* 297(6653), pp. 883–887.

Wald, N.J., Rodeck, C., Hackshaw, A.K., Walters, J., Chitty, L. and Mackinson, M. 2003. First and second trimester antenatal screening for Down's syndrome: the results of the Serum, Urine and Ultrasound Screening Study (SURUSS). *Journal of Medical Screening* 10(2), pp. 56–104.

Wald, N.J., Stone, R., Cuckle, H.S., Grudzinskas, J.G., Barkai, G., Brambati, B., Teisner, B. and Fuhrmann, W. 1992. First trimester concentrations of pregnancy associated plasma protein A and placental protein 14 in Down's syndrome. *British Medical Journal* 305(6844), p. 28.

Wilson, B. 1999. Shifts in mental health policy. In: Hancock, L. ed. *Health Policy in the Market State*. Sydney: Allen and Unwin, pp. 247–264.

Wright, D. 2011. *Downs: The History of a Disability*. Oxford: Oxford University Press.

Yang, Q., Rasmussen, S.A. and Friedman, J.M. 2002. Mortality associated with Down's syndrome in the USA from 1983 to 1997: a population based study. *Lancet* 359(9311), pp. 1019–1025.

Chapter 3

Hands-off work

The following four chapters outline the key findings of my study. The first two explore how screening for Down's syndrome is organised and performed in Freymarsh and Springtown. Specifically, in this chapter, I show how the practices through which Down's syndrome screening is organised contribute to it being 'downgraded'. I define downgrading as practices which denigrate and minimise the importance, value, and reputation of someone or something. Through an analysis of classification and ordering work, I capture how screening is routinised and downgraded as a trivial, non-prioritised task in the organisation of clinical life in three interrelated ways.

Down-grading

First, the task of doing Down's syndrome screening, at least initially, is relegated from consultants to midwives and sonographers. As Down's syndrome screening is viewed as polluting consultants' technical world and the purity of the clinic, this work is 'handed down' and reassigned to non-consultants who are not always officially trained in the practice. Second, professionals implicitly and explicitly define screening, both inside and outside consultations with parents-to-be, as a routine affair. This is accomplished in social processes (e.g. describing screening as a 'simple test') and materials (e.g. the use of doors and rooms). Third, midwives and sonographers classify Down's syndrome screening consultations as a dull, repetitive, and valueless task that does not permit the performance of an authentic professional role. I show how many professionals invest value in tasks which provide them with a chance to become well acquainted with parents-to-be. Since Down's syndrome screening does not offer the opportunity for 'hands-on work', it is constituted as 'hands-off work', that is, a depersonalised and banal task that is not a clinical priority. In short, by examining what professionals *do* and *how* they work, together with analysing the interaction chains of people, objects, and contexts (May and Finch 2009), I uncover how Down's syndrome screening is downgraded and, in turn, routinely embedded and stabilised in prenatal care. Such claims have clear crossovers with my arguments in Chapter 4.

Two points of clarification are required here. First, this downgrading is more common in Freymarsh than Springtown. At Springtown, parents-to-be are offered an appointment time. Only one sonographer and one nurse work during a shift so professionals do not have the opportunity to prioritise one procedure over another. Whilst they certainly value some working practices over others, this rarely manifests itself in practice. As such, the majority of my claims in this chapter concern Freymarsh (the NHS clinic). Second, to be clear, I am not laying the blame for the downgrading of Down's syndrome screening exclusively at the feet of professionals. It is simplistic and offensive to conclude that professionals deliberately, and relentlessly, downgrade screening. The professionals at Freymarsh and Springtown are conscientious, work tirelessly at difficult and complex tasks, and are committed to the cause of parents-to-be. The ongoing classifications of screening for Down's syndrome are, therefore, mostly attributable to the organisation of healthcare and how professionals, positioned in certain ways, are frequently victims of various pressures, not least time restrictions. Their work, in turn, is inhibited and patterned according to each institution and the various negotiations, routines, and stipulations enacted in the clinic (Timmermans and Berg 1997).

The practice of Down's syndrome screening

In Freymarsh, Down's syndrome screening is located, for the most part, in the antenatal department (FAD). The first interaction parents-to-be have with FAD is when attending a 'booking clinic' around ten weeks into a pregnancy. This involves a community midwife performing a dating ultrasound scan[1] and providing parents-to-be with information on prenatal screening and aspects of pregnancy management including but not limited to alcohol intake, exercise, and the consumption of folic acid. It is at this point parents-to-be are offered screening for Down's syndrome and a range of diseases including HIV,[2] syphilis,[3] hepatitis,[4] and rubella[5] (I return to the categorisation of Down's syndrome with 'diseases' later in the book). Parents-to-be who accept Down's syndrome screening in Freymarsh, around 65% according to Dr Karman (FMD consultant),[6] will return to the department around six weeks later to undertake the quadruple screen.

On entry to the department, parents-to-be approach the reception desk, account for their visit, and are told to take a seat before being collected by midwives or maternity care assistants (MCA) depending on their care trajectory. Before moving to the seating area, the receptionist asks parents-to-be to hand over their red folder (given to them by a professional when they first visit FAD) containing personal and physiological details, screening leaflets, and pregnancy management information on, for example, diet and travel safety. The folder is collected by an MCA who delivers it to a trolley holding a blue box. The blue box is positioned directly in front of the midwifery office door so that midwives can notice a folder once delivered. Folders, as material extensions of parents-to-be, are collected by a midwife who, on reading the details inside a folder, determines which professional should meet with parents-to-be and the timing/immediacy of their appointment. Once midwives collect a folder, the respective parents-to-be are summoned to one of five rooms, each a short walk from the waiting area and midwifery office. Parents-to-be who accept Down's syndrome screening are invited by a midwife into a small room to discuss the finer details of the procedure. The small room contains a two-piece sofa, three plastic chairs, a desk, and a computer. Chairs are commonly occupied by a midwife and parents-to-be with the sofa, set against the back wall, occupied by myself and occasionally children. After a midwife describes the procedure and gains consent for screening, parents-to-be are led into a different room where a nurse extracts blood from the arm of a mother-to-be. It is here, according to FAD midwives, where Down's syndrome screening is 'done'.

Parents-to-be at Springtown (privately funded clinic) book a nuchal translucency ultrasound scan (referred to hereafter as 'NT scan'), usually ten to eleven weeks into the pregnancy following a dating ultrasound scan, by telephone. Appointments are logged by administrative professionals who offer an appointment slot and notify parents-to-be of other ultrasound scans available at Springtown. Around twelve to fourteen weeks into a pregnancy, parents-to-be attend Springtown antenatal department (SAD) for an NT scan. After alerting professionals of their presence, parents-to-be are told to sit in the waiting area. If parents-to-be are waiting for a long time, they are offered drinks and an apology by the nurse. Parents-to-be are eventually collected by a nurse, or occasionally the sonographer or myself, who leads them into the clinic. After having their blood withdrawn, mothers-to-be enter the ultrasound room – often alongside partners and other family members – to undertake the procedure. A sonographer sits on one chair and the mother-to-be is invited to lie on the bed with a partner, if present, commonly sitting on the remaining chair. Family members and/or friends can stand beside the bed. Paper towels are placed around the abdomen of the mother-to-be, ultrasound gel is applied, and the sonographer switches on the large television screen connected to the ultrasound machine. This produces a larger image of the womb for parents-to-be and others to see as the sonographer focuses on the smaller monitor. A sonographer describes the procedure, measures the anatomical features of the foetus, and explains that a result will be delivered in a few days. Once more, sonographers acknowledge SAD as primarily where Down's syndrome screening is 'done'.

Hand me Down's[7]

The modern hospital is a complex organisation in which the work of medicine is distributed to different people and across departments. This is certainly true in the case of pregnancy and childbirth, which have been increasingly medicalised in the twentieth century as part of the obstetrics project. Responsibility for much of this care has been seized by (technical) consultants from (non-technical) midwives. Whilst twentieth-century obstetrics concerned itself initially with what it categorised as pathological births, it slowly colonised the entire process of pregnancy by perceiving mothers-to-be as abnormal and defining pregnancy as inherently pathological, that is, a crisis requiring intervention (Hiddinga and Blume 1992). Although midwives reclaimed aspects of pregnancy and childbirth following backlashes about this increasing intrusion, others suggest that the (male) appropriation and medicalisation of pregnancy, rooted in a patriarchal model centuries in the making, persists today (Cahill 2001).

So what about Freymarsh and Springtown? Who performs what care, and particularly Down's syndrome screening, and why? As Star (1995: 3) asks, 'who is doing the dishes? Where is the garbage going?' Previous research identifies how screening for Down's syndrome is carried out by midwives, doctors, or midwives and doctors interchangeably rather than genetic counsellors. In Freymarsh, Down's syndrome screening belongs to a midwife. If parents-to-be receive a lower-risk result as a result of screening, this is confirmed via a letter with no further screen or test recommended. If receiving a higher-risk result, they are invited into the FAD by telephone for counselling with a midwife. In Springtown, Down's syndrome screening is primarily the role of sonographers. Delivering news of a lower-risk result for Down's syndrome to parents-to-be by telephone is the duty of administrative staff with no medical education or training. For a higher-risk result, counselling is done via telephone by a nurse (Francine)[8] or by a specific administrative staff member (Bethan).

In Freymarsh and Springtown, consultants' involvement in Down's syndrome screening is mostly limited to performing subsequent diagnostic tests (amniocentesis/CVS) and managing parents-to-be with previous pregnancy complications. In short, parents-to-be are shifted from the antenatal departments at Freymarsh and Springtown to FMD at Freymarsh if a medical 'problem' is suspected, such as those with a higher-risk result for Down's syndrome following screening and who subsequently consent to diagnostic testing. Whilst Springtown is not officially affiliated with FMD, parents-to-be who have had an NT scan, received a higher-risk result for Down's syndrome, and consented to diagnostic testing are referred to FMD because they are not required to pay for the procedure and they are still under the care of the same consultant as in Springtown (Dr Karman). During a conversation with Springtown (SAD) administrative staff, they explain to me why sonographers, not consultants, are assigned the task of screening for Down's syndrome via an NT scan:

> GARETH: So how do you decide who does the NT scans?
> DOMINIQUE: It's just one of the sonographers.
> HANNAH: Whoever it is who works on that day does them.
> DOMINIQUE: But we usually do them on Fridays and Saturdays when Dr Karman isn't working.[9]

JULIANA: Everyone wants Dr Karman for their NT scans but we don't want to clog up Dr Karman's clinic with NTs and all that easy stuff. Dr Karman does Care Package clients too.

When asked how they decide to allocate NT scans, the SAD administrative staff suggest they are delegated to the days that a sonographer (and so not Dr Karman) is working. This allocation of care is based on a reluctance to 'clog up Dr Karman's clinic with NTs and all that easy stuff', the classification of 'easy stuff' translating to tasks not requiring Dr Karman's expertise. The efforts of Dr Karman are better placed elsewhere in taking charge of cardiac scans, diagnostic testing (amniocentesis and CVS), and 'Care Package clients', namely parents-to-be paying for certain ultrasound scans and counselling sessions (Care Package clients commonly have earlier pregnancy complications, such as recurrent miscarriages).

In Freymarsh, the task of carrying out Down's syndrome screening consultations is similarly demoted to midwives or, more accurately, the 'couch'. In an interview, Lois (FAD midwife[10]) describes a couch's function when discussing her daily work:

> I like doing hands-on midwifery with women because sometimes in clinic, you can be in the office doing results, you can be answering phones, and you're not doing much midwifery. One of the job roles that we do when we have an antenatal clinic is when the midwife is a couch, so they will do what the doctor wants like stretch and sweeps[11] or discuss things with the women and do CTGs.[12] It's hands-on midwifery work I like doing. The prepping for the clinic – its paperwork which is essential because it runs a lot smoother – but it's not what I feel part of what is a midwife's job and there's a lot of admin work involved. I don't think we're being utilised enough and they could be getting more admin staff in who could do that and release us a little more.

The term *couch* is both a noun (a piece of furniture) and a verb. To *couch* something is to arrange, to place and situate in a particular way. Lois defines the couch as someone who performs various duties on demand and who contributes to the arrangement and placing of certain tasks in the hospital. The role of the couch includes, in Lois' own words, 'discuss[ing] things with the women', roughly translating as conducting consultations in which pregnancy information is communicated to parents-to-be (including screening for Down's syndrome). FAD midwives are allocated roles including a 'couch' and working with doctors in a 'specialist clinic', roughly defined as consultations whereby they interact with parents-to-be with specific pregnancy concerns. FAD speciality clinics include breastfeeding, haematology, substance misuse, diabetics and thyroids, asylum seekers, cardiac issues, twin pregnancies, HIV, and recurrent miscarriages.

The specific roles, or temporal identities, of a couch and specialist clinic midwife, among others, are displayed on a whiteboard in FAD. To some extent, work allocation is an unremarkable feature of midwives' practice, yet they are artefacts that make work visible and represent a valuable resource in a chaotic and shifting setting (Allen 2015). The whiteboard reflects a Taylorist distribution of tasks in which professionals are allocated to particular roles; the role of the couch, in turn, extends to what is commonly described by midwives as 'doing a Down's', namely conducting consultations in which Down's syndrome screening is explained to parents-to-be. As midwives rotate their primary job between each shift, they take on the role of couch at different periods of time and, according to Nancy, 'it is the couch's duty to do the Down's'. If a couch – what Nancy calls a 'sort of second hand woman' – is absent (i.e. if they are performing another task), the duty of conducting a Down's syndrome screening consultation falls essentially to any midwife who, as Nancy says, is 'free to do it'. This lack of formality in delegating responsibility for screening consultations is reflected in the following exchange between Lois and Susan (FAD midwives):

> Camilla, Rita, Lois, and Susan (midwives) are in the office. Camilla and Rita are exchanging stories of today's 'misses'.[13] Two red folders have been waiting in the blue box for ten minutes. Lois turns to Susan:
>
> LOIS: Susan, are you free to do a Down's?
> SUSAN: Yes, no problem.
> LOIS: There's another one after as well. I know you're not couch but Lindsay (FAD midwife) is busy doing a scan at the moment. Can you do that one too?
> SUSAN: Yes that's fine.

Camilla and Rita overlook the presence of two red folders (indicative of two parents-to-be attending clinic for Down's syndrome screening) to discuss miscarriage cases. Since Lindsay, the 'couch', is occupied with other tasks, Lois asks Susan if she would 'do a Down's' despite not being ascribed the couch role. Susan accepts this since she is currently liberated from other tasks, a common trend in FAD where calls of 'who is free to do a Down's?' and 'there's a Down's in the box if anyone's available' are regularly heard in the office. Dingwall and Murray (1983: 143) describe how in accident and emergency departments, 'bad patients' are 'detained until there is sufficient slack for the doctor to attend to them'. Whilst parents-to-be who opt to undertake Down's syndrome screening are not ascribed the status of bad patients, per se, they are similarly 'filtered' by midwives under 'a rule of clinical priority' (1983: 144). On a number of occasions, clinical tasks such as counselling parents-to-be following a miscarriage, or even discussing miscarriage cases as Camilla and Rita do in the extract above, took priority over doing screening consultations. Additionally, structural changes in FAD towards the end of my fieldwork led to greater uncertainty about who was conducting screening consultations. The following extract illustrates how this ambiguity played out:

> Eve, Rita, and Camilla (midwives) are completing paperwork in the office. Camilla tells me that she is 'way behind on the bookings for my breastfeeding speciality clinic':
>
> CAMILLA: I'm the afternoon couch but I'm going to be very busy. I doubt I'll have the chance to even do the Down's.
>
> After completing paperwork, Camilla leaves the office to attend to another matter. Jennifer (MCA) enters with a red folder:
>
> JENNIFER: I've got a Down's and I have no idea who is doing them at the moment. There's a few just waiting there to be collected.
> EVE: [Curtly] Well I'm not doing them today.
> RITA: I have no idea who is supposed to be doing them actually.
>
> Frustrated, Jennifer leaves the room and returns the red folders to the blue box. She leaves to find a midwife to carry out the consultation. Eva and Rita debate who should perform this task:
>
> EVE: Camilla is too busy so she can't do them obviously.
> RITA: Shouldn't it be Toni or Emma (midwives)?
> EVE: It should be Toni doing them if Camilla's not around. What is she doing otherwise? Where has she been?
>
> Eve and Rita return to their paperwork. The folders are not attended to for another ten minutes.

Camilla's claim that she may not have a chance 'to even do the Down's' implies that screening consultations are done in a restricted timeframe. In addition, they are implicitly framed as being unworthy of her time which is, it seems, better allocated elsewhere by preparing '[her] breastfeeding speciality clinic' and performing other duties. In response to Jennifer's irritation about who is '[doing] a Down's' (midwives usually collect red folders but MCAs occasionally remind them that there are folders awaiting collection), Eve and Rita distance themselves from this role by attributing accountability for it to Toni. Many hospitals encounter situations not conforming to ideals of best practice, mostly owing to professionals being overloaded with cases. With 'imperfect events' dominating daily routines, organisational ideals can be jeopardised and professionals may relinquish such ideals to be 'realistic' or 'practical' (Emerson and Pollner 1976: 252). In Freymarsh, and particularly with reference to the exchange above, the sheer chaos and demanding nature of hospital life ensures that particular tasks are prioritised over others. Down's syndrome screening, it appears, is heavily implicated in this.

In Springtown, the notion that screening consultations can be done 'on a whim' is essentially impossible since only one sonographer works a shift. Yet the following extract between Sophie (SAD sonographer) and Mr and Mrs Brown (parents-to-be) reveals how Down's syndrome screening can be performed on demand:

Mr and Mrs Brown attend clinic for an early pregnancy scan.[14] During the scan, it transpires that the foetus is twelve weeks and five days old, not eleven weeks and six days old as Mr and Mrs Brown thought. This means that the pregnancy is at enough gestation to undertake an NT scan:

SOPHIE: If you want, we can do the NT scan now [Mr and Mrs Brown look surprised and seem unsure]. The reason I say this is because if you have to book another appointment, you might be too late to do the NT scan since we need to do it before fourteen weeks really. They both cost the same.

MRS BROWN: I think you can just do it now, right [turns to Mr Brown]?

MR BROWN: That's fine by me.

SOPHIE: [Sophie starts measuring the NT] That looks lovely and small.

MRS BROWN: Is that a good sign then?

SOPHIE: Yes.

MRS BROWN: What about my bloods then?

SOPHIE: We can do them today if you want. I'm just going to take the measurements because baby is lying perfectly for it so it makes sense to do it now [Sophie measures the NT which is 1.52mm]. That's lovely and small. That means it will come back as a lower-risk [for Down's syndrome] based on the scan alone. Obviously we match that with the bloods and stuff though and this gives you a result. But based on the scan, it's good news [Mr and Mrs Brown smile]. You've got an active baby in there.

MR BROWN: At least one of them is!

MRS BROWN: Thanks love!

Since the pregnancy dates were recorded incorrectly, Sophie offers Mr and Mrs Brown the opportunity to screen for Down's syndrome instead of having the 'consented-to' early pregnancy scan given the week of gestation and the equivalent monetary cost. After consenting to the NT scan, Mr and Mrs Brown are reassured that they have received a lower-risk result owing to a 'lovely and small' measurement, the former teasing the latter towards the end of the scan about her alleged lethargy during the pregnancy (the significance of humour is explored in Chapter 4). Here, performing a procedure without delay and without parents-to-be necessarily receiving any information about it unwittingly accomplishes the downgrading of screening and the reduction of its value as a medical procedure. It is hard to imagine (and I did not observe) that a more invasive or complicated procedure would merit such casualness about its execution.

Training practices

This downgrading of Down's syndrome screening is further reflected by how midwives and sonographers are taught to perform this task. Interestingly, learning to do Down's syndrome screening was mostly the product of lay pedagogy rather than any mode of structured and formal training. Knowledge production is seen as tacit, embodied, and passed on from knowledgeable professionals to untrained professionals. This corresponds to what Gail (FAD midwife), during one conversation, describes as 'see one, do one'. This occurrence suggests that an observation of a solitary consultation qualifies a midwife for performing this role independently once a similar case presents itself in clinic. Such encounters become vocabulary lessons in which professionals gain knowledge of the specific vernacular for these consultations.

However, the little attention paid to officially training professionals in Down's syndrome screening consultations downgrades its importance. Training to do this particular work, indeed, is a non-priority. In addition, only a few FAD midwives received training in delivering a higher-risk result for Down's syndrome, yet they are ascribed primary responsibility for this care. Midwives are often eager to attend consultations in which parents-to-be receive a higher-risk for Down's syndrome (either in-person or by telephone, but preferably in-person) to learn how to, in short, 'do' this care. The following extract illustrates one such occurrence:

> Terri, Susan, Maggie, and Rita (midwives) are in the office. Angela (midwife) enters:
>
> ANGELA: We've got a higher-risk [for Down's syndrome] in today. Who can do a higher-risk?
> SUSAN: I've never done one but I'm happy to do it.
> ANGELA: OK. Well is it Terri or Rita who have done the higher-risk before?
> RITA: I can do it [Rita collects the folder from Angela].
> MAGGIE: Can I sit in on the phone call Rita? I've never done one before.
> SUSAN: Me too.
> RITA: Bloody hell, I'll have an audience [laughs]. Yes that's fine, girls. The risk factor is 1:17 so the woman shouldn't be too surprised anyway because of her age. I'll call her in twenty minutes as I have some other work to do and the woman might not answer until after nine [a.m.] anyway.

Both Susan and Rita volunteer to 'do a higher-risk', a consultation in which parents-to-be are told they have received a higher-risk result for Down's syndrome following their screening test. Parents-to-be have to be notified of this appointment by telephone, hence Maggie's request to 'sit in on the phone call' since she has not previously been privy to this. Here, higher-risk consultations seem to represent a task which is highly valued, a duty contrasting with the treatment of routine screening consultations. However, with few FAD midwives receiving training in delivering a higher-risk result and little resources being dedicated to this practice, Down's syndrome screening is also subsequently accomplished as a downgraded practice. The following interaction between Sophie (SAD sonographer) and Isobel (SAD nurse) after an NT scan underscores one of the major issues this lack of training can provoke:

> Isobel and I are in the bloods room. Mr and Mrs Sutton (parents-to-be) leave the ultrasound room. Mrs Sutton is crying and Mr Sutton looks upset. They leave the clinic:
>
> SOPHIE: I had a bad feeling about that one. As soon as I saw it on the screen, I thought there was a chance she had miscarried and she had.
> ISOBEL: Poor girl.
> SOPHIE: It's really bad for the girl as it's Friday and now she's got the whole weekend knowing this news before she can talk to anyone. I'm not qualified to discuss this with her and her partner and neither is Isobel.
> ISOBEL: No.
> SOPHIE: This is why it's problematic to have NT scans on the Friday. I feel bad with miscarriages because we just give them a form and send them on their way.

After the Suttons learn of a miscarriage, Sophie bemoans the 'problematic' nature of organising NT scans before a weekend, resulting in her 'just [giving] them a form and [sending] them on their way'. Here, Sophie is 'stepping out of a routine', implying that the 'correctness of the action needs to be explicitly renegotiated' (Berg 1992: 171). Sophie has to account for her non-routine conduct (of allowing parents-to-be to leave the clinic without anyone '[discussing] this with [Mr and Mrs Sutton]'). She further criticises the organisation of care since she is unqualified to discuss the miscarriage with Mr and Mrs Sutton, yet has been assigned the duty of carrying out NT scans for parents-to-be. The demotion of Down's syndrome screening down the clinical hierarchy, a hierarchy reproduced precisely by these practices, to midwives and sonographers triggers profound affects for both themselves and for parents-to-be, whilst also further downgrading the importance and regard of the procedure in prenatal care.

The constituting of classes

Such practices correspond to what Latimer (1999: 179) calls the 'constituting of classes', referring to how patients are categorised into a hierarchy of values that constitute a moral order. Here, particular patients – positioned at the bottom of this order – have their problems refigured from the 'medical' into the 'social'. This reclassification and (re)production of hierarchies of value means that patients are discharged or made 'disposable' (Latimer 1997: 176) since they do not belong to the technical terrain of medicine. Disposal, for Berg (1992) and Latimer (1997), refers to how professionals engage in a mode of ordering which helps them keep their world in order and square accounts to themselves and others. For Latimer, shifting a patient's identity does not mean disposing of people but, rather, part of their responsibility to certain patients so they can care for those with whom they feel compelled to work. This constituting of classes, in turn, is what helps keep the medical domain in order.

This constituting of classes is also evident in Freymarsh and Springtown. In the extracts above, it is clear how Down's syndrome screening is figured as a trivial procedure that can be performed on-demand and as a non-prioritised task in the hierarchy of clinical value (shown not least by its relegation down the professional pecking order). It is 'easy stuff' which 'clogs up' the precious time of consultants since parents-to-be undertaking Down's syndrome screening, at least in the early stages, have yet to attain the status of clinical interest (Bosk 1992). There is a moral division of labour (Hughes 1971) in which those of higher status and professional standing specialise in desirable cases whilst concurrently shifting the undesirable work 'to others with less standing' (Emerson and Pollner 1976: 243). Since Down's syndrome screening consultations do not promise 'the speedy resolution of organic problems', the 'special skills' of doctors are reallocated to contexts in which they can be put to 'much greater use' (Strong 1979: 225). Although falling under the remit of obstetric care, screening is relegated by consultants to midwives, thus establishing their territory and protecting the purity of the clinical space by consigning the polluting work of screening down the division(s) of labour. Screening consultations, as such, become downgraded as non-technical tasks which represent 'trivia' (Dingwall and Murray 1983: 144) or 'matter out of place' (Douglas 1966: 36) in obstetric care until diagnostic testing (amniocentesis or CVS) is required, namely, when screening becomes diagnostic.

'We do normality, we don't do pathology'

As well as screening being downgraded via its relegation down the clinical hierarchy, as described above, it is downgraded further through professionals' classification of this particular practice. In Freymarsh and Springtown, midwives and sonographers regularly describe Down's syndrome screening as a routine and expected component of a pregnancy trajectory. Speaking of her impending exit from FMD[15] during one conversation, Elena (FMD head midwife) claims:

> There's just more misery walking through the door every day. I've had enough. I'll go back to FAD to do the ordinary stuff. It'll be nice to go back to that as I've done it all before.

Elena accounts for her imminent departure from FMD as relating to 'more misery walking through the door every day'. Relocating to the FAD, for Elena, represents a return to the 'ordinary stuff'. This classification of 'ordinary stuff' parallels Dr Karman's (FMD consultant) distinction during one conversation between the 'routine stuff' of the FAD and the 'weird stuff' of FMD, the latter referring to treating and managing certain foetal 'defects'. In Freymarsh and Springtown, Down's syndrome screening is categorised as routine and ordinary stuff, a mundane component of prenatal life. A routine refers to a set of actions 'repetitively carried out with a certain automatism' without explicitly reflecting on or legitimating the actions involved (Berg 1992: 170). The routine of Down's syndrome screening, by interconnecting with the routines of other tasks in both Freymarsh and Springtown, can be classified as what Nancy (FAD midwife),[16] in the following extract, defines as 'normality':

> Rosie (MCA) and Nancy are in the office. Nancy is on the telephone to Mrs Earl who is part of Nancy's specialist clinic for twin pregnancies. The conversation ends. Nancy turns to me:
>
> NANCY: [Mrs Earl] is having a real rough time of it at the moment. Her feet, legs, and thighs have swollen massively. She's only a petit lady so it looks terrible. Her skin around there is rock hard too. I just hope it isn't anything serious like preeclampsia.[17] I recommended she should see someone. I said to her 'I'm a midwife, I'm not a doctor'. But I would feel awful if I didn't say anything and then something happened to her or the baby. It doesn't sound right, does it? It does happen to women but at what point does it become pathological, you know? We do normality, we don't do pathology. Doctors do all the oedema,[18] preeclampsia, and stuff. I'm not medical but that worries me, you know, is it physiological or pathological? Can you imagine what would happen if I didn't say anything?
>
> ROSIE: You'd get in a lot of trouble!
>
> NANCY: That's my official licence gone. And I couldn't live with myself if something happened. Some of the women we have are a bit precious and demand our care but at the end of the day, you understand it because they want their babies to be healthy and who wouldn't?

Unsure when Mrs Earl's problems 'become pathological', Nancy downplays her professional competence by deferring authority to doctors who 'do all the oedema, preeclampsia, and stuff'. Importantly, Nancy claims 'we do normality, we don't do pathology'; distancing herself from 'medical' and 'physiological or pathological' matters, she worries that a failure to 'say anything' would constitute both an emotional burden and potential loss of employment. Since Mrs Earl does not integrate into the category of normality, she is referred to a doctor.

However, since Down's syndrome screening is performed by midwives, it is not classified as pathological or meriting doctors' intervention. Positioned as unproblematic and 'normal', screening consultations fall to midwives dealing with 'normality', that is, to borrow Dr Karman's term, the 'routine stuff'. This framing of Down's syndrome as a routine practice and non-technical matter often manifests itself in screening consultations. Toni (FAD midwife), for instance, describes the consultation to parents-to-be as 'just a chat', whilst Tara (FAD midwife) and others frequently describe the procedure to parents-to-be as a 'simple blood test'. The following fieldnotes are taken from a consultation between Lois (FAD midwife) and Mrs Patel (mother-to-be):

LOIS: Today we're going to chat about the Down's syndrome test. Have you had Down's syndrome screening before?

MRS PATEL: Yes.

LOIS: Do you understand it then?

MRS PATEL: I just had it last time, I didn't know anything about it. I wasn't told I was having it and I was just told that nothing is good news.

LOIS: OK. So do you know much about Down's syndrome and effects it has?

MRS PATEL: Yes.

LOIS: Well this is a blood test which doesn't affect the baby. You're provided with a lower-risk or higher-risk result. A lower-risk result means no further testing but it doesn't mean the baby definitely doesn't have Down's syndrome. The screen has a 70% detection rate and if you're lower-risk, you receive a letter saying this within ten working days. A lower-risk result can be 1 in 200 or something like 1 in 1,000. The cut off is 1 in 150. So anything above that is a higher-risk and you'd get that within five working days so it's done quite quickly. You'd be offered an appointment within twenty-four hours and we'd offer you an amniocentesis where we check the fluid around the baby. It has a miscarriage rate, though, of 1 in 100. But if you do have a higher-risk result, we invite you in and we have a good chat about what you want to do about it. Have you thought about what you would do? Would you want to know whether you're a lower-risk or higher-risk?

MRS PATEL: Yes I want to know.

LOIS: OK.

Lois fills in Mrs Patel's medical record. Lois leads Mrs Patel to another room for the quadruple screen.

After Mrs Patel accounts for her lack of knowledge regarding Down's syndrome screening ('I just had it last time, I didn't know anything about it'), Lois accepts Mrs Patel's claim that she knows about the condition itself (I return to knowledge of the condition in Chapter 5) and provides information constituting the staple diet of Down's syndrome screening consultations: its non-invasiveness, the production of a lower-risk or higher-risk result, the source and timeframe of news, the prospect of diagnostic testing, confirming that parents-to-be want to undertake screening, and the accuracy of the procedure (admittedly the latter point is rarer). Defining screening consultations as 'simple' or 'a chat' reflects how midwives and sonographers constitute Down's syndrome screening in everyday clinical life and how this downgrades it, arguably, as an unproblematic practice. Framed as a simple procedure, its value is downgraded. This can explain why parents-to-be consent to screening, naturalising and normalising what is supposed to be an *opt-in* rather than *opt-out* practice (Tsouroufli 2011).

The routinisation of Down's syndrome screening is also reflected in the material and spatial organisation of prenatal care. Earlier, I referred to how structural changes in FAD caused confusion regarding who carried out screening consultations. This confusion also translated to the location of such consultations. When asked who carries out screening consultations (and where) following such changes, Camilla (FAD midwife) claims:

> We haven't really figured that one yet! The couch starts doing Down's, then they come over to clinic [with doctors], and then they do some clinic stuff [with doctors]. I don't think any of us know about it. It changes every week and we just end up doing them in whatever room we can get.

Camilla identifies how the couch, as previously defined, initially does consultations until 'clinic stuff' takes priority. In contrast, Down's syndrome screening is not allocated, at least at this moment, a permanent home for carrying out consultations – nor is repairing this viewed as a priority. This lack of prioritisation is reflected in FAD by folders, on many occasions, resting in the blue box whilst other clinical tasks took priority. The blue box and red folders, in such instances, remain symbolic and are mobilised in ordering who or what is deserving of primary attention. This material treatment of Down's syndrome screening, both through folders remaining in boxes for extended periods and consultations not being assigned a stable home, indicates a lack of prioritisation and disposes of the procedure as non-urgent. The following fieldnotes were taken during a morning at Freymarsh:

> I enter the office. Lindsay, Lois, and Rita (midwives) are busy at their desks. Lois is today's couch:

LOIS AND LINDSAY: Good morning!

GARETH: Morning! How are you both doing?

LINDSAY: All good.

LOIS: Good thanks. You?

GARETH: Good thanks. I was told yesterday you've got ten consultations for Down's syndrome screening today, Lois. Is that right?

LOIS: [Looking surprised] Really? I'll check but I haven't received any yet.

Lois leaves the office and returns from reception smiling with four folders in her hand. It is 09:15 and there were appointments at 08:00, 08:10, 08:20, 08:30, 08:40, 08:50, 09:00, 09:10, 09:30 and 10:00. It later transpires that two consultations were carried out by another midwife. Lois leaves the office to collect the next appointment.

It is in such situations that Down's syndrome screening is disposed of as a non-priority, as a trivial duty performed by the couch or unattached, with other tasks becoming prioritised in the organisation of care. In addition, consultations are performed, as Camilla described in an earlier extract, 'in whatever room we can get'. The importance of both materiality and spatial arrangements in healthcare work has been explored elsewhere in a small but important body of literature (Allen 2015; Bromley 2012; Fannin 2003; Fox 1997; González-Santos 2011; Latimer 2013; Martin et al. 2015; Prior 1988; Rawlings 1989; Sandelowski 2003; van Hout et al. 2015; White et al. 2012). Clinics are places where people, objects, technologies, and talk intersect and interact, that is, they are sites of material and discursive construction. The scenery and 'props' of settings (Goffman 1959) mediate the practices, experiences, and interactions of people working or visiting the clinic – and can either facilitate or impede how care is enacted.

Both Freymarsh and Springtown are occupied by many materials. This includes more 'obvious' artefacts such as technical equipment (e.g. ultrasound machines), computers, sofas/chairs, and tables but also more 'mundane' materials such as folders, leaflets, posters, whiteboards, and obstetric calculators.[19] Focusing on Freymarsh, the attention, or not, to the significance of materials and space in the delivery of care (e.g. doing screening 'in whatever room we can get') is reflected during a consultation between Toni (FAD midwife) and Mr and Mrs Hayes (parents-to-be):

Mr and Mrs Hayes enter the room and sit on the chairs. Toni follows them into the room. The door is left propped open by a bin:

TONI: So are you OK?

MRS HAYES: Yes but I've seen so many different midwives. I'm so confused.

TONI: Well today you're seeing me for your Down's syndrome screening. So you know this does not provide a yes or no answer?

MRS HAYES: It's just the blood test, yes?

TONI: Yes. Your result has to be a 1 in 150 result or less to be considered higher-risk and so be offered an amniocentesis.

MRS HAYES: So the figure has to be 1:151 or above for me to get away with it and 1:149 or less to not get away with it?

TONI: Yes.

MRS HAYES: So a higher-risk can be a 1 in 150 or 1 in 2 then?

TONI: Yes. If you're higher-risk, we contact you and invite you into clinic. If you're lower-risk, we send you a letter telling you this.

MR HAYES: So the letter is for good things and the phone call is for bad things?

TONI: Yes. If you're higher-risk, we call you in 3–4 working days but if you don't hear anything, this is a good thing.

Toni takes some details about future prenatal bookings and asks Mr and Mrs Hayes if they have more questions. Toni leads Mr and Mrs Hayes to the bloods room for their quadruple test.

Toni tells Mrs Hayes that she will be screened for Down's syndrome today, later providing information on the outcome of the procedure and the possibility of diagnostic testing should a higher-risk result be established. Mr and Mrs Hayes seem to desire and distinguish binaries in their accounts, with risk factors amounting to '[getting]' or 'not [getting] away with it' and contact being established in the case of either 'good things' or 'bad things'. Whilst Toni does not seek reassurance from Mr and Mrs Hayes that they wish to undertake screening, an action encouraged by many midwives at Freymarsh (i.e. the notion that parents-to-be can opt out of the procedure should be reiterated), the importance of the door being propped open during the consultation highlights the informality and routine-ness of screening consultations. For Berg (1992: 171), routines 'facilitate medical action' and 'supply a framework which delineates what is proper action and what is not'. Such routines are not just social categories but are also 'materialised'; routines do not just dictate the use of an instrument or form but the form itself structures an interaction and becomes an 'integral [part] of the routines' (1992: 171). What is shown here is how Down's syndrome screening is trivialised and, so, routinised via interweaving social and material elements.

Importantly, this shifts in FMD. Here, much more attention is paid to materials and spatial arrangements, with the space being inscribed with symbolic meaning by professionals. Consider the following fieldnotes from a consultation between Dr Karman (FMD consultant) and Mr and Mrs Parnell (parents-to-be):

I follow Dr Karman into the room. As I enter, Elena (FMD head midwife) is sitting with Mrs Parnell. Dr Karman asks me to close the curtain.

Mr and Mrs Parnell have previously been notified about a foetal heart defect. Dr Karman tells Mr and Mrs Parnell that whilst the defect is 'manageable', the baby requires surgery after childbirth and delivery at another hospital better-equipped to handle the case is recommended. Elena leaves the consultation and ensures the curtain remains closed.

This contrasts with the following fieldnotes from a consultation between Dr Karman and Mr and Mrs Fitz (parents-to-be):

Dr Karman and I enter the consultation room. The door and curtain remain open. Dr Karman sits next to Mr and Mrs Fitz who have just had an ultrasound scan after a suspected problem:

DR KARMAN: I have good news. The testing you underwent revealed there's nothing wrong with your baby.

MR AND MRS FITZ: [Breathe sigh of relief] Thank you.

DR KARMAN: There are no underlying structural problems which have been detected via ultrasound so in my opinion, there is no indication of any form of abnormality.

MRS FITZ: Oh, that's great news.

MR FITZ: Yes, thank you doctor.

DR KARMAN: I'm glad it's good news. Now you can go and enjoy your Christmas!

MR FITZ: Definitely.

MRS FITZ: Uh-huh.

Interestingly, during a consultation with a positive outcome, Dr Karman makes no effort to ensure that the door or curtain are closed. In contrast, on other occasions where a diagnosis or suspected diagnosis is provided, there is frequently an active effort to ensure that curtains and/or doors are closed. Dr Karman also reflected on the spatial dimensions of care in a conversation we had in the early stages of fieldwork:

Dr Karman leads me to a large room, telling me it is dedicated to performing an amniocentesis or CVS as well as other procedures. Dr Karman explains parents-to-be are later invited back to FMD should a diagnosis be established and then shows me the room where this news is delivered. The room is large containing a desk, three chairs, and a bed:

DR KARMAN: The room for delivering the news is much bigger than we used to use. It was the size of a cupboard. Now when you're delivering news of this nature, that's inappropriate isn't it?

In the first extract, Dr Karman and Elena ensure that the door and curtains remain closed during the consultation. In her study of a maternity unit,

Burden (1998) captures how women position curtains to invite attention or refute it. Similarly, in FMD, professionals use curtains and doors to deliver *good care* (the second extract, though, highlights how this attention to materiality is not always needed in accomplishing good care). In the third extract, Dr Karman highlights the inappropriateness of a room that is 'the size of a cupboard' when 'delivering news of this nature'. In FMD, FAD, and SAD, care is a social and material achievement, with the materiality of the space often being conducive to the nature of the consultation. By asking 'what buildings do' (Gieryn 2002) and what they – and the materials contained in them – 'perform' (Stephens et al. 2008), I show how the materiality of Freymarsh and Springtown not only demarcates divisions of labour (e.g. through folders, the whiteboard) but also signifies privacy and what constitutes serious, or more trivial, matters. In the case of Down's syndrome screening, whilst doors are not always propped open during consultations, such an incident is indicative of its downgrading in the clinic.[20] Positioned lowly in a hierarchy of clinical priorities and classified as 'just a chat' or 'simple test', it is upheld as a routine component of prenatal care.

'Hands-on midwifery work'

So far, I have described how professionals do not always prioritise Down's syndrome screening in their daily work. Other research has shown how patients are subjected to categorisation processes, demarcating the appropriateness of their presence in the clinic, which can lead to some patients being seen before others (Becker 1993; Timmermans and Berg 1997; Hillman 2007; Jeffery 1979; Latimer 1999; Dingwall and Murray 1983; White et al. 2012). Whilst moral and critical appraisals of patients in FAD and SAD are rarely observed, certain tasks are preferred and, thus, prioritised. This highlights another way in which the organisation of prenatal care downgrades Down's syndrome screening, namely, by routine screening consultations being cast as mundane and tedious duties. The classifications of un/desired roles are highlighted during a conversation with Lisa (SAD sonographer) about her imminent shift at Freymarsh[21]:

> LISA: I've got my kidneys, gall bladders, and livers now. I hate them. I spent the morning doing prenatal stuff but we change it up so I'll be stuck doing them now.
> GARETH: So you don't like them?
> LISA: You just don't enjoy them as much. It's not pregnancy stuff. It's boring, you know? Instead I'm going to be doing all of the yuk stuff [laughs].

Lisa prefers the 'pregnancy stuff', as a more enjoyable component of her daily routine, over 'the yuk stuff', translating to patients who have problems with their kidneys, gall bladder, or liver. We can return here to the distinction made by Lois (FAD midwife) cited earlier between 'hands-on midwifery work' against tasks which she says do not reflect 'part of what is a midwife's job'. So what kind of work is 'hands-on midwifery work' compared to tasks which are not 'part of what is a midwife's job'? Whilst Lois includes the task of 'discuss[ing] things with the women' as normal midwifery, small acts of separation – often 'buried in habit' (Douglas 1966: 9) – are made within this more condensed network of professional tasks. Down's syndrome screening, in turn, frequently falls short of being hands-on midwifery work. Consider how Lindsay (FAD midwife) describes Down's syndrome screening consultations during an interview:

> [Consultations] are repetitive. [...] I wouldn't say it was boring but it does get a bit repetitive. You're just providing information.

Similar to Lindsay, other midwives and sonographers describe Down's syndrome screening consultations as dull and routine, a pedestrian part of their working practice. For Lindsay and others, this stems from the repetitive nature of consultations because their care is limited to providing factually correct medical information. During a conversation, Esther (SAD sonographer) tells me:

> I get bored of saying the same thing over and over. You have to try and make it sound different and interesting every time. It's like a performance. [...] The difficulty is sometimes you're saying the same thing over and over again. Sometimes you can't remember whether you've said certain things or not, so it absolutely is a performance. It does become routine. And you've got be very careful that it doesn't come across to the women that you're [screening] which is why I couldn't do it day in, day out.

Esther claims that she is 'bored of saying the same thing over and over', identifying the professionals' labour in ensuring the 'performance' of a 'routine' procedure is never fully revealed. The tedium cited by Esther is reflected in the following fieldnotes taken from a consultation between Jackie (FAD midwife) and Mr and Mrs Wotton (parents-to-be):

> JACKIE: Let me weigh you first [Mrs Wotton is weighed]. Are you here for the Down's syndrome screening?
> MRS WOTTON: Yes.
> JACKIE: Do you know that you're not going to find anything from this test? It is only going to tell you whether your baby has a high or low chance of Down's syndrome.
> MRS WOTTON: Yes.
> MR WOTTON: Yes, that's all in the information anyway.
> JACKIE: OK. Amniocentesis will be offered if you come back as a higher-risk. The cut off here is 1:150 which means if you're 1:150 or higher, you're a higher chance.

MRS WOTTON: So if it's higher than 1 in 150, that means I have a high chance?

JACKIE: Yes. With the amniocentesis, a needle is put in the stomach and this takes out some fluid which is sent to the labs and this can say whether your baby is affected. Do you have any more questions?

MR AND MRS WOTTON: No.

Jackie fills in some details on the medical record. She takes Mrs Wotton to the bloods room to have the quadruple screen. I return to the office. As I write up notes, Jackie enters the office. Angela (midwife) is working at another desk:

JACKIE: [Turning to me] You can sit in with me on more [consultations] if you want. You'll get bored of hearing the same thing over and over eventually. It gets repetitive and boring after a while. The brain shuts down and the mouth starts playing when doing Down's syndrome screening!

ANGELA: Yes [laughs]!

The 'repetitive and boring' nature of screening consultations, Jackie quips, gives rise to 'the brain [shutting] down and the mouth [starting] playing'. A similar sentiment is expressed by the administrative staff at Springtown who describe themselves as 'parrots' and 'like recorded messages' (Hannah, SAD administrative staff) when providing information about Down's syndrome screening, signifying the rudimentary and anodyne nature of communicating information about the procedure.

Professional identity-work

In the context of this study, one reason why Down's syndrome screening is seen as boring and routine is because it is not part of the highly valued hands-on midwifery work vital for performing a meaningful professional identity (here, I understand identity as never unified/singular and as collectively constructed across diverse and intersecting discourses, practices, and contexts at different moments). This is vital for FAD midwives since midwifery in its entirety, according to Elena (FMD head midwife), is 'a Cinderella of the whole antenatal service', with 'the big guns up on the delivery suite'. Elena highlights how some aspects of prenatal care are professionally impure and regularly promise a low intra-professional status. Some midwives claimed that they 'bear the brunt of complaints' (Francine, FMD head midwife) and doctors do not receive the same negative treatment that they experience, attributing this to 'the doctor midwife psychology'. During one exchange, Amy (FAD midwife) suggests that 'other departments don't actually get that midwifery is a really important part of antenatal care' whilst Rita (FAD midwife), after I asked her during one conversation how her day was progressing, answered 'understaffed, underpaid, and working with new systems that no-one knows how to follow!'

Although Rita's complaint was light-hearted, it reflects other complaints of midwives and sonographers. In his study of genetic counsellors, Bosk (1992) refers to such professionals as a 'mop-up service' (1992: 57) who perform undervalued and low-esteem work deferred by higher-status colleagues. This mostly involves managing the emotional toils of parents-to-be in the context of reproductive decision-making. In the context of my research, I loosely adopt the term 'mopping up' to refer to the work of professionals, and parti-cularly midwives, to capture how they felt they occupied a lower status in the clinical hierarchy and were positioned as 'gatekeepers without turf' (1992: 72), meaning they had to carry out the tasks which were undervalued in prenatal care (not always related to emotional placation, as in Bosk's research). Although professionals did not always self-identify as being a mop-up service, constructing and retaining a meaningful professional identity was of para-mount importance for midwives – particularly since they commonly viewed their role as undervalued. Hands-on midwifery work provides crucial material for this construction. Asked about her job roles, Susan (FAD midwife) explains:

> You do a lot of screening, a lot of deciding if people are higher-risk or lower-risk pregnancies, you do speciality clinics which are really inter-esting like diabetics, anti-D clinic, and rheumatology clinics. There are loads of positives working in FAD. [...] I'm not a fan of looking at blood results, checking them off, and sending out letters. I feel like it's a waste of a midwife's role. But I like doing my haematology clinic because I get to know my women as well. Because they're such high-risk women, we work quite a lot together and if they get any problems, they can call me.

Susan describes the positives of working in FAD together with the less desirable roles of 'looking at blood results, checking them off, and sending out letters'. She defines the latter tasks as 'a waste of a midwife's role' whilst conveying her enjoyment of her haematology speciality clinic. On a number of occasions, FAD midwives claimed ownership over their own speciality clinics which are valued as enjoyable tasks appropriate for identity-work. Susan's enjoyment stems from '[getting] to know my women', claiming ownership over 'high-risk women' who she is able to establish a relationship with. Lindsay (FAD midwife) similarly identifies the opportunity to help parents-to-be and 'sort out their problems' as one major component in for-mulating a meaningful identity. Camilla (FAD midwife) likewise claims that she likes speciality clinics since 'you get to know women and their case'. During one conversation, Francine (FMD head midwife) describes how she would not want to work in FAD since her role in FMD involves 'more rewarding work':

We all have our own areas of interest. I don't like kidneys. They don't interest me very much. But I like everything else. They're a bit, it sounds awful, but a bit common and mundane. I like the cases that you can actually feel that you're offering the families support and advice so they can get some benefit, however hard the decision they're making is. Whether it is to continue or not to continue [a pregnancy], they feel they've got someone to turn to. It's a really nice feeling to be able to do that. It is very satisfying, which I don't really get as much in normal midwifery because if it's normal, a lot of women just go through pregnancies and don't really need extra support. I like to feel more useful really.

Francine suggests that professionals have their own areas of interest; she says kidneys are 'a bit common and mundane' whilst she places value on care which offers embodied opportunities of '[feeling] more useful' and 'offering the families support and advice' that are absent in 'normal midwifery'. This highlights how professionals embrace tasks providing them with an opportunity to help and work in a manner they view as integral to their professional status. During an interview, Sophie (SAD sonographer) similarly describes her preference for undertaking 'tough cases' which offer a chance to 'reassure' parents-to-be if 'things are not going to plan'. Similar to Sophie's classification of 'bad things', translating roughly to tasks tendering a space for professionals to help parents-to-be, Gail (FAD midwife) describes cases in which 'there is not a good outcome' as 'interesting':

These make the work a little bit more interesting if you like than where you've got the run of the mill stuff. When you've got some things a little bit more out of the ordinary, it can make it a little bit more interesting, can't it? We all need variety and if you're doing the same things day after day, you can get a little bored or it can get a little samey.

Gail crafts a distinction between the 'interesting' work which offers 'variety' and the 'run of the mill stuff' which breeds boredom and is 'a little samey'. Such tasks often translate to encounters that professionals define as 'emotional'. When asked about her job during an interview, Elena (FMD head midwife) explains:

It is a very emotional job. I'm not saying you don't get involved with patients but when you're delivering bad news to someone, there's another ten women out there and you've got to do exactly the same thing with them. The unthinkable is a reality here and it relates to a lot of stuff that happens in [FMD]. [...] It's challenging for you and it's challenging for the parents. [...] I always make a point of not wearing my uniform when I leave for home and it was a little change I did. Because I used to take the emotions of the work home but then, I did that sort of very physical thing of taking the uniform off and putting my clothes on before going home. Because a lot of it is protecting yourself as well as sort of giving the information. [...] There are still times that you still get stuck up on some patients but I think we're all human. It's natural.

In an environment in which 'the unthinkable becomes a reality', professionals must adopt tactics to manage this 'emotional job'. Elena suggests that her uniform sustains a physical barrier between work life and home life. Whilst Elena's role is in FMD, a department in which 'bad news happens' (Francine, FMD head midwife), many professionals in FAD and SAD also claimed that they had self-protecting strategies for preserving emotional distance from their work. Gail (FAD midwife), for instance, suggests developing 'a dark or black sense of humour' as a 'way of coping'. In addition, professionals claim that in order to avoid undermining the principles of professionalism, they have to 'be detached from patients in some respects' (Rita, FAD midwife) and 'draw the line and still be a professional' (Martha, FAD midwife) even if it is 'hard to switch off' (Susan, FAD midwife).

The 'emotional labour' (Hochschild 1983) involved for professionals in healthcare institutions (Kerr 2013; Larson and Yao 2005) and midwifery specifically (Deery 2009; Hunter 2004) has been reported elsewhere. However, by considering what tasks professionals define as 'emotional' accomplishments, I show how they – whilst difficult in many respects – are highly valued by midwives and sonographers and considered as an important component of becoming a competent professional. Far from being impersonal or disinterested actors, the professionals' labour is frequently 'an emotional and an affective labour too' (Fitzgerald 2013: 133). They have an emotional investment in their work and, whilst attempting to claim distance, establish an 'affective commitment' (Fitzgerald 2013: 136). In Freymarsh and Springtown, duties that afford the professionals an opportunity to invest in, help, and 'get to know' parents-to-be are frequently those that are preferred and prioritised in the clinic. Down's syndrome screening does not tender that prospect.

Professionals do not build a relationship with parents-to-be during screening consultations because the latter commonly attend the clinic only on one occasion, and because consultations are frequently conducted in a short timeframe. Pressured to maintain patient flow according to organisational logic (Allen 2015), professionals may not always have the time to dedicate to certain procedures. Others have identified the conflict between the time professionals have to explain Down's syndrome screening and the time required to fully discuss the procedure (Ahmed et al. 2013; Sooben 2010; Williams et al. 2002). During a conversation, Esther (SAD sonographer) describes the difficulty of conveying 'empathy' within a restricted encounter:

You can't show empathy during some procedures because you've only got ten minutes to do the scan and people get annoyed because when other people have problems which take up time and the clinic's run over time, how can you possibly give compassionate care if you're constantly thinking my time with patients is going to overrun?

In FAD and SAD, the timeslots allocated for quadruple screens and NT scans are ten minutes and twenty minutes respectively (although this is negotiable, as Esther demonstrates above when claiming that 'you've only got ten minutes to do the scans'). Consultations rarely extend beyond this time period yet their premature conclusion is much more common. In FAD, more time is dedicated, for example, to counselling parents-to-be who experience a miscarriage in the current pregnancy and to managing parents-to-be attending speciality clinics. In SAD, more time is dedicated, as another example, to performing cardiac ultrasound scans as opposed to NT scans. Within time-restricted encounters, then, the capacity to invest in parents-to-be by establishing 'patient contact' (Amy, FAD midwife) and 'sort[ing] out their problems' (Lindsay, FAD midwife) is not possible.

This is not exactly the 'dirty work' described by Hughes (1971) or Emerson and Pollner (1976) in that the professionals in Freymarsh (and Springtown, to some extent) do not explicitly classify screening as 'shit work' (Emerson and Pollner 1976: 243) or as disgusting, degrading, or shaming. Nor does this work involve acting in opposition to the desires or needs of parents-to-be (of doing something *to* clients). Yet professionals often lament Down's syndrome screening as being boring, repetitive, and hands-off work that provides little opportunity for *doing* (authentic) midwifery and doing something *for* parents. Professionals have a clear conception of what tasks closely resemble the ideal or symbolic work of their profession – and what tasks may be labelled a nuisance and imposition (Hughes 1971). Down's syndrome screening, as a time-restricted and (assuming professionals' language) *unemotional* task, is seen as hands-off work and, as such, is further downgraded in the clinic.

Summary

This chapter, in sum, captures how Down's syndrome screening is organised and, in turn, downgraded in three ways that re-accomplish its status as a routine affair. First, screening is relegated from consultants to midwives and sonographers who are not always officially trained in the practice. Since it pollutes consultants' technical world, screening is reclassified as belonging to the realm of midwives and sonographers who 'mop-up' (Bosk 1992) the mess. Though Bosk claims that professionals have work shifted onto them because of a pre-existing medical hierarchy, I suggest that this hierarchy is repeatedly re-accomplished through the classification and subsequent non-prioritisation of Down's syndrome screening. Categorising screening, at least initially, as a non-technical matter that does not belong to obstetrics protects the purity of obstetric care. Through this constituting of classes (Latimer 1999), thus, Down's syndrome screening is used as a resource for reproducing divisions between professionals and their tasks – and is downgraded as such.

Second, Down's syndrome screening is downgraded through being constructed as a simple and routine component of prenatal care accomplished in both social processes and cultural materials. FAD midwives highlight how their work is concerned with 'normal' rather than 'pathological' (or technical) care. However, so much of midwives' daily routines involve surveillance and monitoring mothers-to-be, such as taking bloods and performing ultrasound scans that arguably contribute to creating a pathological pregnancy. This relation between everyday ('normal') midwifery work and Down's syndrome screening shows how the latter is entangled in 'motility', referring to how people or things are moved in different spaces of discourse which invokes specific effects by altering the very essence of such entities (Latimer 2007; 2013; Latimer and Munro 2006). In the case of Down's syndrome screening, professionals switch discursive domains to recognise how, in one moment, screening is a downgraded assignment (counselling parents-to-be before the procedure) but, in another moment, is upgraded work when it gets 'serious' (a higher-risk result requiring counselling). Yet in many ways, screening occupies a liminal space; it is often not valued or deemed worthy of FAD midwives' primary attention, and yet it is relegated from FMD consultants for whom it is not yet clinical enough to merit attention. Down's syndrome screening is emplaced in midwifery and sonography yet, concurrently, it does not become their primary professional concern (at least in midwifery). As such, it becomes downgraded and refigured as a routine and expected component of prenatal care.

Third, in their ordering work in the clinic, midwives and sonographers reproduce classifications which, in turn, cast Down's syndrome screening as a familiar character in their daily drama. It is positioned as a repetitive, trivial, and non-prioritised task which is not part of hands-on midwifery work, that is, it is not part of their domain of expertise. FAD midwives, occupying a space in which they are asked to perform a wide range of duties, 'attach to' (Latimer 2013) and invest value in tasks that are 'emotional', such as delivering news of a miscarriage or helping parents-to-be experiencing a different but equally serious setback, and that afford them an opportunity to become acquainted with parents-to-be; a 'steady flow of interesting cases with sufficient time to savour each one', then, is favoured (Dingwall and Murray 1983: 143). Parents-to-be are often the raw material for professionals' identity construction and performance of competence. Down's syndrome screening, owing to its monotony and incapacity to regularly offer the rewards identified above, is not suitable for their identity-work and self-understanding; it is not 'real midwifery' and, subsequently, is accomplished as a downgraded practice. In Chapter 4, I extend this analysis to illuminate how Down's syndrome screening is further configured as a routinised practice.

Notes

1 A dating scan is an ultrasound scan occurring around eight to fourteen weeks into a pregnancy. The scan is used to check how many weeks pregnant a mother-to-be is, whether it is intrauterine, whether it is viable, and whether it is a multiple pregnancy. Sonographers will also check the ovaries for cysts. Parents-to-be often receive a picture of the imaging at the end of the scan.

2 HIV (human immunodeficiency virus) is a virus that causes the acquired immuno-deficiency syndrome (AIDS). It attacks the immune system, allowing opportunistic infections and cancers to thrive.

3 Syphilis is a sexually transmitted bacterial infection which mothers-to-be can pass onto a foetus.

4 Hepatitis is a condition defined by liver inflammation and characterised by inflammatory cells in the tissue of an organ.

5 Rubella is a viral infection. It is usually a mild condition but can be more serious during a pregnancy.

6 As a reminder, many professionals working at Springtown also work at Freymarsh. However, the reference to Freymarsh or Springtown in parentheses is used to signify where I observed the vast majority, if not entirety, of each respective professional's work. As an example, Dr Karman is a consultant in both Freymarsh and Springtown but was observed most frequently in the Freymarsh foetal medicine department (FMD). Hereafter, I use FMD when referring to the Freymarsh foetal medicine department.

7 Hand me Down's is my own term. It is a play on Down's syndrome and the idiom 'hand me down' which refers to how something is passed on to one person after being discarded by another person.

8 Francine is also an FMD midwife. FMD is where I observed her working life most frequently.

9 This also explains why many of the extracts cited in this book involve Esther (SAD sonographer). Whilst other sonographers (Olivia, Lisa and Sophie) also per-form NT scans during their shifts, Esther often works on Friday and Saturday when many NT appointments are allocated. This means that Esther conducts a large amount of NT scans during her shifts. Heather (sonographer) was not trained in NT scans but was trained in 4D scans (more on this later in the book).

10 Lois is also an FMD midwife but I observed her most frequently in FAD.

11 A stretch and sweep, also known as membrane sweeping, is a technique of labour stimulation.

12 Cardiotocography (CTG) is a technical means of recording foetal heartbeat and uterine contractions in pregnancy. This is typically performed in the third trimester.

13 Misses is a term used by professionals to refer to parents-to-be who have had a miscarriage in their pregnancy.

14 An early pregnancy scan is an ultrasound scan performed between seven and eleven weeks of a pregnancy to confirm the number of foetuses, the presence of a heartbeat, the size of a sac/foetus, and the possible presence of internal bleeding.

15 As a reminder, FMD is a referral service. In the context of Down's syndrome screening, parents-to-be are only referred to FMD from FAD if they decide to pursue diagnostic testing. This is where CVS or an amniocentesis is performed, where parents-to-be will be counselled about a result, and where parents-to-be can have a termination of pregnancy if requested.

16 Nancy is also an FMD midwife but I observed her most frequently in FAD.

17 Preeclampsia is a condition characterised by high blood pressure and a large amount of protein in the urine of a pregnant woman. It affects up to 10% of

pregnancies and severe cases develop in 1–2% of pregnancies. Although most cases of preeclampsia cause no problems and improve soon after a baby is delivered, there is a risk of serious complications affecting both the mother and her baby.

18 Oedema is the medical term for fluid retention in the body.

19 An obstetric calculator is designed to help professionals assess when pregnant women are due to deliver.

20 The routinisation of Down's syndrome screening is also reflected by my relatively smooth access to consultations. With consent, professionals and parents-to-be almost always accepted my presence without objection. Practices categorised as 'serious' or 'invasive' (e.g. diagnostic testing, trans-vaginal ultrasound scanning), in contrast, required a more active engagement with issues surrounding my entry. This further elucidates how Down's syndrome screening is downgraded as a routine and mostly straightforward procedure for which I am granted entry.

21 Lisa works in both SAD and the Freymarsh radiology department. Our conversation follows an interview which was organised during her lunch break at Freymarsh.

Bibliography

Ahmed, S., Bryant, L.D. and Cole, P. 2013. Midwives' perceptions of their role as facilitators of informed choice in antenatal screening. *Midwifery* 29(7), pp. 745–750.

Allen, D. 2015. *The Invisible Work of Nurses*. London: Routledge.

Becker, H.S. 1993. How I learnt what a crock was. *Journal of Contemporary Ethnography* 22(1), pp. 28–35.

Berg, M. 1992. The construction of medical disposals: medical sociology and medical problem solving in clinical practice. *Sociology of Health and Illness* 14(2), pp. 151–180.

Bosk, C.L. 1992. *All God's Mistakes: Genetic Counseling in a Pediatric Hospital*. Chicago: University of Chicago Press.

Bromley, E. 2012. Building patient-centeredness: hospital design as an interpretive act. *Social Science and Medicine* 75(6), pp. 1057–1066.

Burden, B. 1998. Privacy or help? The use of curtain positioning strategies within the maternity ward environment as a means of achieving and maintaining privacy, or as a form of signalling to peers and professionals in an attempt to seek information or support. *Journal of Advanced Nursing* 27(1), pp. 15–23.

Cahill, H.A. 2001. Male appropriation and medicalization of childbirth: an historical analysis. *Journal of Advanced Nursing* 33(3), pp. 334–342.

Deery, R. 2009. Community midwifery 'performances' and the presentation of self. In: Hunter, B. and Deery, R. eds. *Emotions in Midwifery and Reproduction*. Basingstoke: Palgrave Macmillan, pp. 73–89.

Dingwall, R. and Murray, T. 1983. Categorisation in accident and emergency departments: 'good' patients, 'bad' patients and 'children'. *Sociology of Health and Illness* 5(2), pp. 127–158.

Douglas, M. 1966. *Purity and Danger: An Analysis of the Concepts of Pollution and Taboo*. London: Routledge and Kegan Paul.

Emerson, R.M. and Pollner, M. 1976. Dirty work designations: their features and consequences in a psychiatric setting. *Social Problems* 23(3), pp. 243–254.

Fannin, M. 2003. Domesticating birth in the hospital: 'family-centred' birth and the emergence of 'home-like' birthing rooms. *Antipode* 35(3), pp. 513–535.

Fitzgerald, D. 2013. The affective labour of autism neuroscience: entangling emotions, thoughts and feelings in a scientific research practice. *Subjectivity* 6(2), pp. 131–152.

Fox, N. 1997. Space, sterility and surgery: circuits of hygiene in the operating theatre. *Social Science and Medicine* 45(5), pp. 649–657.

Gieryn, T. 2002. What buildings do. *Theory and Society* 31(1), pp. 35–74.

Goffman, E. 1959. *The Presentation of Self in Everyday Life*. London: Allen Lane.

González-Santos, S.P. 2011. Space, structure and social dynamics within the clinical setting: two case studies of assisted reproduction in Mexico City. *Health and Place* 17(1), pp. 166–174.

Hiddinga, A. and Blume, S.S. 1992. Technology, science, and obstetric practice: the origins and transformation of cephalometry. *Science, Technology and Human Values* 17(2), pp. 154–179.

Hillman, A. 2007. *Negotiating Access: Practices of Inclusion and Exclusion in the Performance of 'Real' Emergency Medicine*. Unpublished Ph.D. Thesis, Cardiff University.

Hochschild, A. 1983. *The Managed Heart: Commercialization of Human Feeling*. Berkeley: University of California Press.

Hughes, E.C. 1971. *The Sociological Eye: Selected Papers*. Chicago: Aldine.

Hunter, B. 2004. Conflicting ideologies as a source of emotion work in midwifery. *Midwifery* 20(3), pp. 261–272.

Jeffery, R. 1979. Normal rubbish: deviant patients in casualty departments. *Sociology of Health and Illness* 1(1), pp. 91–107.

Kerr, A. 2013. Body work in assisted conception: exploring public and private settings. *Sociology of Health and Illness* 35(3), pp. 465–478.

Larson, E.B. and Yao, X. 2005. Clinical empathy as emotional labour in the patient–physician relationship. *Journal of the American Medical Association* 293(9), pp. 1100–1106.

Latimer, J.E. 1997. Giving patients a future: the constituting of classes in an acute medical unit. *Sociology of Health and Illness* 19(2), pp. 160–185.

Latimer, J.E. 1999. The dark at the bottom of the stairs: participation and performance of older people in hospital. *Medical Anthropology Quarterly* 13(2), pp. 186–213.

Latimer, J.E. 2007. Diagnosis, dysmorphology, and the family: knowledge, motility, choice. *Medical Anthropology* 26(2), pp. 97–138.

Latimer, J.E. 2013. *The Gene, the Clinic and the Family: Diagnosing Dysmorphology, Reviving Medical Dominance*. London: Routledge.

Latimer, J.E. and Munro, R. 2006. Driving the social. *The Sociological Review* 54(S1), pp. 32–53.

Martin, D., Nettleton, S., Buse, C., Prior, L., and Twigg, J. 2015. Architecture and health care: a place for sociology. *Sociology of Health and Illness* 37(7), pp. 1007–1022.

May, C., and Finch, T. 2009. Implementation, embedding, and integration: an outline of normalization process theory. *Sociology* 43(3), pp. 535–554.

Prior, L. 1988. The architecture of the hospital: a study of spatial organisation and medical knowledge. *British Journal of Sociology* 39(1), pp. 86–113.

Rawlings, B. 1989. Coming clean: the symbolic use of clinical hygiene in a hospital sterilising unit. *Sociology of Health and Illness* 11(3), pp. 279–293.

Sandelowski, M. 2003. Taking things seriously: studying the material culture of nursing. In: Latimer, J.E. ed. *Advanced Qualitative Research for Nursing*. Oxford: Blackwell, pp. 185–210.

Sooben, R.D. 2010. Antenatal testing and the subsequent birth of a child with Down syndrome: a phenomenological study of parents' experiences. *Journal of Intellectual Disabilities* 14(2), pp. 79–94.

Star, S.L. 1995. Introduction. In: Star, S.L. ed. *Ecologies of Knowledge: Work and Politics in Science and Technology*. Albany, NY: State University of New York Press, pp. 1–35.

Stephens, N., Atkinson, P. and Glasner, P. 2008. The UK Stem Cell Bank as performative architecture. *New Genetics and Society* 27(2), pp. 87–98.

Strong, P. 1979. *The Ceremonial Order of the Clinic: Parents, Doctors and Medical Bureaucracies*. Henley-on-Thames: Routledge and Kegan Paul.

Timmermans, S. and Berg, M. 1997. Standardization in action: achieving local universality through medical protocols. *Social Studies of Science* 27(2), pp. 273–305.

Tsouroufli, M. 2011. Routinisation and constraints on informed choice in a one-stop clinic offering first trimester chromosomal antenatal screening for Down's syndrome. *Midwifery* 27(4), pp. 431–436.

van Hout, A., Pols, J. and Willems, D. 2015. Shining trinkets and unkempt gardens: on the materiality of care. *Sociology of Health and Illness* 37(8), pp. 1206–1217.

White, P., Hillman, A. and Latimer, J.E. 2012. Ordering, enrolling, and dismissing: moments of access across hospital spaces. *Space and Culture* 15(1), pp. 68–87.

Williams, C., Alderson, P. and Farsides, B. 2002. Dilemmas encountered by health practitioners offering nuchal translucency screening: a qualitative case study. *Prenatal Diagnosis* 22(3), pp. 216–220.

Chapter 4

A can of worms

In Chapter 3, I explored how Down's syndrome screening is downgraded in different but interrelated ways. This chapter extends this focus by identifying two ways in which screening for Down's syndrome is further sedimented as a routine part of prenatal care. First, the entangling rhetoric of 'informed choice' and 'non-directive care' – so prevalent and popular in reproductive practices – constitutes a resource that allows professionals to 'dispose' (Berg 1992; Latimer 1997) of Down's syndrome screening and allocate full responsibility for decision-making to parents-to-be. By focusing on how professionals draw on discursive grounds and rules to legitimate and 'account' for their conduct (Garfinkel 1967), I also explain how this rhetoric is used by professionals to quash their own concerns and unease with screening.

Here, there exists a contradiction between frontstage official accounts that professionals are expected to convey and their private misgivings about the seriousness of Down's syndrome as a health condition, the negative implications of giving risk factors to parents-to-be, the extent that parents-to-be can make truly 'informed' choices, and the 'eugenic' quality of prenatal screening for the condition. Behind the mundane and mechanical nature of this technical procedure, there is a significant social and moral agenda, and staff subsequently engage in serious emotional labour in order to provide 'informed' choice. Yet this care obligation – to reallocate decision-making to parents and provide clinically accurate information without any bias or intervention – lets professionals detach themselves from decision-making with regards to screening whilst, at the same time, playing a key role in shaping it. This produces circumstances in which screening is downgraded and, in turn, naturalised as a 'normal' pregnancy practice.

Second, Down's syndrome screening is routinised by parents-to-be, often with the sonographer, focusing largely on the 'social' rather than 'medical' dimensions of ultrasound. The social rituals of undertaking an ultrasound scan – obtaining pictures, inviting family and friends to 'meet' the baby, and recreating family narratives – figure screening for Down's syndrome, carried out in Springtown (but not Freymarsh) using ultrasound technology, as routine and expected conduct for parents-to-be. Professionals' imperative to merge providing medical information with a consumer-friendly performance implicitly and inadvertently trivialises Down's syndrome screening and downgrades its value as a medical procedure.

'It has to be your choice'

I begin this chapter by identifying how 'informed choice' (or 'informed consent') and 'non-directive care', transposable discourses infiltrating Down's syndrome screening and prenatal care more generally, are enacted in the clinic and what this accomplishes. Notions of choice and autonomy are at the heart of current biomedical discourse in the UK and beyond. In recent years, there has been a shift in healthcare systems in the global North from an intensely paternal medicine to an informed choice model (Mol 2008; Williams et al. 2002a), reflecting a departure from impersonal 'corpse care', of clinicians treating the body mechanically as a silent and docile object with personal markers stripped away, to individualised 'consenting care' in which the responsibility of decision-making is usually assigned to patients. This 'logic of care' (Mol 2008) places an emphasis on looking and listening to 'grant patients their life as well as knowing them as if they were dead' (Mol and Law 2004: 44). In a broader and more egalitarian view of (holistic) care, patients are to be considered as individuals with a right to participate in decisions. Reproductive technologies, in particular, are heralded as a route to liberation since they offer parents-to-be information about, and control over, offspring (Kerr and Cunningham-Burley 2000), though this may not always be empowering (Lippman 1994; Shakespeare 2011).

One way for understanding how professionals define informed choice and non-directive care with respect to screening is to examine the information provided to parents-to-be and what details are omitted from consultations (Bosk 1992). In a setting in which the enactment of bureaucratic regulations transforms work into a distinct ceremonial order (Strong 1979), one must attend to how policy is translated and gets talked into practice, and how it is enrolled, enacted, or deferred by professionals during interactions with parents-to-be. In Freymarsh and Springtown, both midwives and sonographers emphasise their alignment with the entwining principles of non-directive care and informed choice when doing Down's syndrome screening. In FAD, parents-to-be are given a multitude of booklets and information on this procedure. One booklet reads:

> Only you can decide whether to have the test or not. Some women want to find out if their baby has Down's syndrome, and some don't. All women are offered a screening test for Down's syndrome but the decision whether to have the test or not is yours. You can discuss with your midwife what you want to do. They will support you whatever you decide.

This booklet, much like similar literature and policy documents, suggests that parents-to-be 'can discuss' procedures with midwives but they are the 'only' ones who can decide about screening. Individual choice is a common rhetorical device in policy frameworks for Down's syndrome screening, focusing on the individual rather than the social context of screening and testing. Professionals claim that they abide by such stipulations, with Nancy (FAD midwife) stressing during one conversation that parents-to-be 'should make their own personal choice and be true to themselves'. I asked Camilla (FAD midwife) during an interview how she defines informed choice:

> Informed choice is giving them as much information as you can, the pros and cons, looking at the whole thing, what the consequences are of having it or not having it and what it'll mean to them. Once you feel you've given the information and they seem to understand what you're saying, and they can give you that back, then I'd say they're making an informed choice. [...] [Parents-to-be] sometimes ask me if many people have the test. So I say 'some people will do this' and try to show them there are different outcomes and you don't have to just say yes or no.

Camilla describes informed choice as 'giving [parents-to-be] as much information as you can', including the dis/advantages and outcomes of screening. She claims that this offers parents-to-be a chance to '[make] an informed choice'. However, her suggestion of telling parents-to-be 'some people will do this' arguably undermines the ideal of informed choice by influencing the decisions of parents-to-be. This is made more explicit elsewhere. In NT scans, for instance, Esther (SAD sonographer) regularly suggests amniocentesis is 'advised' if a higher-risk result for Down's syndrome is established. Esther's comments, intended or not, can undercut the principle of informed choice. Describing amniocentesis as 'advised' arguably does not allow for an autonomous 'choice', advice being translatable to subtly disciplining parents-to-be into making certain choices. Advice, then, can be explicit (Silverman 1987; Strong 1979) or implicit (Latimer 2007; Pilnick and Zayts 2012). However, as Schwennesen and Koch (2012: 283) note, undercutting the rhetoric of informed choice does not *always* translate into bad practice. Whilst not always immediately compatible with the non-directive ethos, professionals' conduct can constitute 'good care' by supporting parents-to-be to make choices that are often on the basis of uncertain knowledge; an example of this can be telling parents-to-be, as Camilla does, that 'some people will do this'. By answering the plea of parents-to-be for some direction, professionals arguably move closer to promising 'informed choice' by supporting them to make a decision. Rather than this being described as a serious problem of oppressive power resulting in coercive moments of decision-making, such actions are categorised as ensuring informed choice since non-directive care may not always be the most suitable response.

Despite Camilla's account showing how policies are made and unmade in everyday affairs, she aligns with definitions of informed choice and non-directive care as defined by other professionals, policies, and booklets. Similarly, Amy (FAD midwife) says during one screening consultation:

> Our job is to give information to make an informed choice. Because it has to be your choice because then you have to live with the choice afterwards.

Professionals convey an image of the 'ideal' (Goffman 1959) professional, he or she who communicates with parents-to-be in a clear and non-directive manner. This is not to say, though, that this is always an easy task. Both midwives and sonographers regularly identify the difficulties of ensuring fully informed choice when screening for Down's syndrome. Sophie (SAD sonographer), for instance, claims that parents-to-be 'will have their own interpretation of the facts'. Along with citing the discrepancies of 'interpretation' between parties and how conveying information to parents-to-be is difficult, Sophie suggests that parents-to-be often solicit advice. In response, Sophie says that her care is limited to '[telling] them the facts' since 'it's an individual decision' and 'I can't tell [parents-to-be] the answer'. A similar sentiment is expressed by many other midwives and sonographers. The purpose of this chapter is not necessarily to assess and disclose whether informed choice or non-directive care are achieved in some capacity (this has, frankly, been done to death within the literature on the social life of reproductive technologies and, in particular, Down's syndrome screening). Rather, attention is given to how professionals reflect on this rhetoric and, in turn, how they use it to account for their conduct and to accomplish certain things in the prenatal setting.

The ambiguities of professionals

Interestingly, in the backstage of interviews or conversations where parents-to-be are absent, midwives and sonographers often recount their own concerns regarding Down's syndrome screening. In various forms of 'communication out of character' (Goffman 1959), professionals 'step out' and convey thoughts that are incompatible with the fostered impression of the 'idealised' professional. The well-understood alignment with promising informed choice and non-directive care sits awkwardly alongside three ambiguities that the midwives and sonographers convey related to screening: (1) quadruple screening is not as accurate as an NT scan; (2) screening is routinised yet can create undue anxiety; (3) screening reflects eugenic purposes as Down's syndrome is clinically categorised as 'compatible with life'. Whilst I discuss the latter concern in Chapter 5, I address the first two reservations here.

Quadruple screening in Freymarsh — as a reminder, screening at Springtown is done via an NT scan — is critiqued by several midwives for its inaccuracy. During one conversation, Maggie (FAD midwife) claims:

It just seems quite a strange test. I wouldn't have it. I might have the nuchal translucency scan. I don't really think the [quadruple] test really tells you anything anyway, does it? You've got your low-risk result so you are low-risk but you can still have your baby with Down's syndrome or you can be high-risk and you can still not have a baby with Down's syndrome. I don't really think it makes much difference in my opinion.

Maggie's concerns are shared by many professionals who quote quadruple screening as approximately 75–80% accurate, meaning that around 75–80% of foetuses with the condition receive a screen-positive result. The NT scan in SAD, in contrast, is quoted as being around 90% accurate. Maggie refers to this when claiming that she 'might have the nuchal translucency scan' (presumably because of its increased accuracy). Much like Maggie, Amy (FAD midwife) says she would not undertake quadruple screening herself, although she is careful to reiterate 'it is an individual choice' and 'my opinion doesn't mean I should influence anyone else not to have the test done'. Eve goes a step further by referring to quadruple screening as 'rubbish' as 'you don't get definite answers', but she says that she would also not reveal this reservation to parents-to-be since 'I can't put my opinion across to someone'.

The accuracy of the screening test is an important point. However, a more common denouncement from professionals concerns how screening, in their view, can needlessly generate anxiety and uncertainty for parents-to-be. As such, I focus on this concern for much of the chapter. Feelings of fear and anxiety among parents-to-be before, during, and/or after Down's syndrome screening have been recognised in previous accounts (Aune and Möller 2012; Burton-Jeangros et al. 2013; Green and Statham 1996; Heyman et al. 2006; Hunt et al. 2005; Ivry 2006; Markens et al. 1999; Marteau 1995; Pilnick et al. 2004; Remennick 2006; Williams et al. 2005). Clarke (1991) argues that the implicit assumption of screening is that parents-to-be will find the resulting information powerful and beneficial. However, this is challenged by Clarke on the premise that it can produce serious dilemmas for parents-to-be, possibly turning them into what Rapp (2000: 3) calls 'moral pioneers'. Much less research has been carried out with respect to how professionals view Down's syndrome screening, although the work of Williams et al. (2002b) shows how they can view screening as limiting women's choices. In Frey-marsh and Springtown, Down's syndrome screening is often classified as what Camilla (FAD midwife), among others, refers to as a 'can of worms':

After a consultation, Camilla tells me that she has thought about what she would do if she 'came back as a higher-risk [for Down's syndrome]':

CAMILLA: Most [parents-to-be] are just like 'oh I'll have [screening] anyway'. I don't think most of them realise it can open up a can of worms. If they're not going to have the amniocentesis if they're a higher-risk result, what's the point in having the test in the first place? Otherwise they're just going to have a worrying pregnancy. I couldn't believe it when I found out that three out of four kids with Down's syndrome came back as a lower-risk result.[1] The lower-risk isn't really that reassuring then is it? It makes you think what is lower-risk?

Camilla expresses her worry that Down's syndrome screening can 'open up a can of worms'. If parents-to-be would not entertain the prospect of agreeing to diagnostic testing if a higher-risk result is established, Camilla questions why parents-to-be undertake screening in the first instance. She also highlights how the production of risk factors, as scientific artefacts, require interpretation and are not just givens ('it makes you think what is lower-risk?') and how parents-to-be undertake screening uncritically and, essentially, without great thought. Susan (FAD midwife) similarly associates the naturalisation of screening, of parents-to-be accepting screening since it is perceived as 'just an extra test so I'll have it done', with a lack of perception among parents-to-be regarding the procedure as possibly having 'huge implications'. This contradicts other research exploring how clinicians/scientists retain cognitive authority and avoid criticisms of their work, thereby marginalising more critical commentaries, by stressing the value of choice and how technologies can prevent certain genetic conditions and diseases (Cunningham-Burley and Kerr 1999). The following extract illustrates this difference:

The consultation is over. It lasted twenty to twenty-five minutes (longer than usual). Mr and Mrs Ingram seemed unclear as to why they attended clinic today and what Down's syndrome screening entails. After they leave, Lois turns to me. She says 'well that was difficult' and laughs whilst shaking her head:

LOIS: The absolute classic is parents having these tests just because they can. Just because they're available, they're like 'I might as well have it'. And they don't really think about what might happen afterwards with these results. They don't think about whether they want an amniocentesis or think they might be a higher-risk. It's a can of worms really. It's the same with other testing as well like HIV, rubella, syphilis, and that. They're like 'oh we might as well'. Well, no, not you might as well! These tests have massive implications. And with the amniocentesis, they can have a full test and discover other things aside from Down's [syndrome].[2] It's a minefield really. If you detect something else, do you tell them? There was a woman last week who had a one in thirteen result for Down's [syndrome]. When we told her that she had a one in thirteen chance, she said 'I just thought I'd come back as a low-risk. Now I don't have a clue what to do'. If people are going to have the test, they should probably know what they'd do with that result afterwards.

Lois claims that the 'classic' is parents-to-be undertaking Down's syndrome screening compliantly 'because they can'. Citing the case of a mother-to-be who received a 1:13 risk factor, she accuses parents-to-be of not considering the 'massive implications' of screening; 'it's a minefield'. Some midwives and sonographers, in their 'treatment of the absent' (Goffman 1959), allege that parents-to-be commonly accept screening uncritically on account of its availability and do not engage with the relevant prenatal literature. They believe that the docile acceptance of parents-to-be, indeed, means they do not consider the potential consequences of their actions (i.e. receiving a higher-risk result and having to decide about diagnostic tests). This is hugely problematic for many professionals because screening and testing can 'discover other things aside from Down's [syndrome]' and so, in turn, 'poses more questions than answers' (Gail, FAD midwife), 'causes a lot of stress' (Francine, FMD head midwife), constitutes a 'slippery slope' (Rita, FAD midwife), and 'alters the course of pregnancy completely and can leave [parents-to-be] in a position of whether or not they want to continue with the pregnancy when initially it started out for them as a simple test for Down's syndrome' (Lois, FAD midwife). By identifying Down's syndrome screening as possibly producing undue anxiety and uncertainty, midwives and sonographers express their own reservations and, arguably, subtly critique it.

Informed choice in everyday practice

I have identified a tension in the accounts of professionals: they express ambiguities and anxieties about screening yet spend much of their day aligning with principles of informed choice and non-directive care, discourses that have constituted key principles of prenatal care for a prolonged period. Personal concerns are suppressed by citing such rhetoric as taking priority in prenatal care. Professionals delivering this programme are encouraged to suspend all values and judgement about how they believe one should behave and how a decision should be made. This is clearly evident in the following fieldnotes taken from a consultation in Freymarsh between Susan (FAD midwife) and Mr and Mrs Payton (parents-to-be), an extract atypical in length (the consultation lasted around 25 minutes) yet typical in its depiction of professionals aligning with the rhetoric of informed choice and non-directive care:

SUSAN: So do you know anything about this Down's syndrome test?
MRS PAYTON: No.
SUSAN: Well if you wish, we can check your bloods today using your age, whether you smoke, the results of the blood test, and your weight to

calculate a risk factor for Down's syndrome. It's not definite in that it won't give you a diagnosis. You'll just be put into a category of higher-risk or lower-risk. A lower-risk result which is a 1 in 150 result or more means you'll get a letter. But it's important to remember that you could have a 1 in 100,000 risk of having a child with Down's syndrome but it doesn't mean the baby definitely doesn't have the condition. It just means there's a 1 in 100,000 chance it will. A higher-risk result is on the other side, so a 1 in 150 or less result. So you could have a 1 in 12 risk or 1 in 30 risk of having a kid with Down's syndrome, for example. But if you do have a 1 in 30 risk, the baby is still unlikely to have Down's syndrome. Do you understand?

MRS PAYTON: Yes.

SUSAN: So if you're higher-risk, an amniocentesis is offered. Do you know about amniocentesis?

MRS PAYTON: Yes.

Susan explicates the finer details of screening after Mrs Payton claims she knows little about it. In many consultations, parents-to-be frequently appeared confused about their presence in clinic ('I can't remember why we're here to be honest'), were unaware of what the procedure entails ('I just said yes for every test'; 'I haven't really thought about it'; 'I don't know about it but my brother and his wife had it so I thought we would have it too'), and had not considered the implications or possibility of diagnostic testing ('so what is amniocentesis?'; 'I don't really know what I'd do but I'll have the test now as I just want to know if something's happened or if something's wrong'). In addition, many decisions to accept screening seemed to be accounted for as a formality in the hope that everything would be well. Nonetheless, in this consultation, Susan explains that Mrs Payton will be 'put into a category of higher-risk or lower-risk' since a diagnosis is not provided and that a lower-risk result does not necessarily translate to not having a child with Down's syndrome. After offering more examples of risk factors, Susan continues:

SUSAN: So would you go on to have an amniocentesis, and do you want the blood test or not? [Mrs Payton hesitates].

MR PAYTON: I would want to know [if the baby had Down's syndrome] but she wouldn't want to do anything so it's pointless even having this test.

MRS PAYTON: Do lots of people have the test?

SUSAN: It depends.

MR PAYTON: I'd have the test if I was a woman.

SUSAN: If you have a higher-risk result and decide not to have an amniocentesis, the result might stress you out for the rest of the pregnancy. You'll spend the rest of the pregnancy worrying [Mr and Mrs Payton pause].

MR PAYTON: It's a catch twenty-two really.

SUSAN: We can only give all of the information and it's up to you whether you decide to have the test.

Mrs Payton appears hesitant to answer after Susan asks whether she would 'go on to have an amniocentesis' and whether she would 'want the blood test or not', with Mr Payton claiming he would 'want to know' yet his partner would 'not want to do anything' (presumably meaning that Mrs Payton would not opt for terminating a pregnancy following a positive diagnosis). It is clear that Mr and Mrs Payton did not previously thrash out the finer details of Down's syndrome screening. Susan's account at the end of the extract involves the first explanation that after '[giving] all of the information', it is 'up to you whether you decide to have the test'. This, however, is supplemented with a warning that a result could 'stress you out for the rest of the pregnancy' (what Mr Payton calls a 'catch twenty-two'). The consultation resumes:

MRS PAYTON: [Turns to Susan] What do you think?

SUSAN: I can't decide for you. An amniocentesis provides a definite diagnosis and means you could either continue or terminate the pregnancy. Obviously the termination would be offered for medical reasons.

MR PAYTON: So it's a personal preference, [Mrs Payton].

MRS PAYTON: [Seems anxious. Turns to Susan] What do you think?

SUSAN: It's your choice. [...]

MR PAYTON: You'll probably be alright, [Mrs Payton]. You're young.

SUSAN: Yes. If you do want the test, you'll have to do it soon as you're already eighteen weeks and four days pregnant and we can't offer the test after about nineteen weeks. Remember the only way you'll know for sure is through amniocentesis. This is only screening today.

MR PAYTON: It's only a blood test, [Mrs Payton].

MRS PAYTON: [After a long pause]: I think it'd be good to know if I was higher-risk. So quite a lot of people have this test?

SUSAN: I don't know the exact statistics but it's a personal choice whether or not to have the test.

Mrs Payton seeks advice by asking Susan once if other mothers-to-be undertake screening, and twice what Susan '[thinks]'. She responds by once more emphasising 'it's a personal choice'. Susan agrees with Mr Payton's claim that Mrs Payton is young so will 'probably be alright' (i.e. it is unlikely that the baby will have Down's syndrome) and claims that a decision needs to be made promptly since the test will not be available soon owing to the current week of gestation. It continues:

MRS PAYTON: [Unsure] There's lots of decisions to be made. It adds stress doesn't it? I'd rather not have it done.

SUSAN: OK. Well you'd probably end up in the lower-risk category anyway with your age and weight.

MRS PAYTON: So what would you do?

SUSAN: I can't say.

MR PAYTON: [Irritated] Love, she's already told you twice that she can't say and it's a personal decision!

SUSAN: Why don't you go for a walk and come back in ten minutes to see what you want to do?

MR AND MRS PAYTON: OK.

Mr and Mrs Payton leave. Susan turns to me and breathes a sigh of relief:

SUSAN: That's why we do these consultations. Otherwise she would have the bloods and not know what they were for.

Mrs Payton returns after one minute without Mr Payton and tells Susan that she will not have the screen.

There are many acts of negotiation taking place here between each person. Mrs Payton tries to enrol Susan in decision-making by emplacing trust in Susan to make the decision for her. This is a trend that emerged in other consultations at FAD. In patient-centred consultations, parents-to-be sometimes seem reluctant to engage in individual decision-making and assume their ascribed role, preferring to defer authority to the 'expert' professional. However, Susan disposes of her responsibility for Down's syndrome screening by broadly referencing the rhetoric of 'choice' and by accounting for her role as solely communicating medically based information about the procedure and its outcomes. This is similar to Springtown, where care is primarily confined within rigid perimeters of giving medically accurate information. Sonographers regularly provide the same account for screening during an NT scan: they say that they are measuring the nuchal translucency, how its enlargement is connected to chromosomal conditions, how this results in the production of a risk factor, and how diagnostic testing can be offered if a higher-risk result is established. In doing so, they avoid primary responsibility for decision-making. Such strategies involve professionals taking comfort in the principle of 'safety in numbers'; their care is appropriate as colleagues do the same and '[normalise] the action as legitimate within their shared universe of meaning' (Scott et al. 2013: 431).

Despite the prevailing ideals of informed choice and non-directive care shaping professionals' accounts and interactions, the practical realities of information provision, moulded by the emergent logic of everyday rituals, deliver an encounter perhaps contrary to professionals' intentions; in the prenatal clinic, the 'messiness of mundane practices fail to submit to theoretical ideals' (Mol 2008: 43). Indeed, the stating of options does not always amount to the neutral provision of advice since some options have the force of a directive (for instance, to draw on an example used earlier, 'advising' an amniocentesis). Professionals' methods of information provision – embedded and consumed in a complex array of medical, political, and social practices and pressures – are likely to influence certain decisions (Browner et al. 1996; Kerr et al. 1998; Lippman 1994; Pilnick 2008; Rapp 2000). Rather than censuring professionals for this, we may ask whether fully autonomous and informed decision-making in the context of Down's syndrome screening can ever exist.

This points to how care is accomplished in the interactions, materiality, and practices of the clinic with decisions made in interdependent relations; care is something you *do* as opposed to something which *is* (Latimer 2000; Mol 2002). At its heart inter-subjective and a matter of process, care is an open-ended and unsettled entity involving the body, emotions, and identity-work, a practice stratified and distributed across time and place that is always achieved and never attributable to an impartial account (Mol 2008). In short, what we regard as choice is never a value-free activity and is always subjected to various influences, few of which are straightforward or transparent. Rather than repeating well-established arguments around how non-directive care and informed choice is/is not achieved in practice, however, I elucidate what this rhetoric accomplishes. Professionals align with this rhetoric and use it as a resource to effectively dispose of screening. Parents-to-be are instituted as rational decision-makers who, provided with clinically correct information, are able to choose between alternative courses of action (Silverman 1987). They are enrolled in, and subjected to, disciplining practices (Foucault 1973) that encourage self-management. Positioned as active decision-makers, parents-to-be are accountable and 'gain autonomy at the cost of being morally responsible for their actions' (Allen 2013: 42). What this means, then, is that by professionals disposing of responsibility for screening and by suppressing their own concerns and ambiguities, it persists as a normal and expected procedure. Parents-to-be are accused of undertaking screening uncritically and without due consideration of possibly imminent complications – yet little is done to repair this organisational fracture. The professionals' disposal of screening, figuratively if not physically, creates circumstances in which it is viewed by parents-to-be as routine. Without knowledge of impending difficulties and professionals' worries, and with all of the clinical information in hand, they 'might as well'.

Language barriers

Professionals' detachment from Down's syndrome screening and reallocation of responsibility are evident in their interactions with parents-to-be whose first language is not English. The toils of communicating information about Down's syndrome screening if the first language of parents-to-be is not English has been reported elsewhere (Ahmed et al. 2013; Hey and Hurst 2003). This is particularly a challenge for professionals in Freymarsh as the hospital serves a large population whose first language is not English. The problems that a language barrier can create are outlined after a consultation between Toni (FAD midwife) and Mrs Garcia (mother-to-be):

> The consultation has ended. Mrs Garcia seemed confused throughout the encounter. After Toni leads Mrs Garcia into another room for the quadruple screen, she returns to the room and says:
>
> TONI: I'm not sure if she understood that. There was a bit of a language barrier.

During the consultation, Toni's objective appears to be providing medically correct information rather than ensuring that Mrs Garcia has fully understood the procedure. In FAD, a translator is not offered, or at least is not immediately available, once undertaking Down's syndrome screening (partners may translate for a mother-to-be, and vice versa). Emma (FMD midwife)[3] tells me, after a similar consultation with a mother-to-be whose first language is not English, that:

> When the woman and the partner are foreign, it makes me a bit uneasy. You have to question whether they really fully understand the information you are giving to them. We get a lot of people in here, some from very different religious backgrounds, and they might not abort the baby because of their religious beliefs. But if they don't speak very good English, they may not know about this screening and if they wouldn't have the amniocentesis anyway, then they may not want screening in the first place. But they may not know about this if they don't understand.

Again, the professionals prioritise providing clinically correct information, consistent with organisational recommendations, over ensuring that this data has been fully comprehended by parents-to-be. Although language barriers are a less common example, it highlights how screening is downgraded in the clinic. It is interpreted as a procedure which does not demand the use of translators for potentially mending splintered interactions. Resources, as important indicators of what patients or clinical tasks are valued, are not allocated here. Instead, care is constricted to tendering clinical information on *what is* as opposed to *what ought to be*. Professionals' anxieties around screening are made absent in everyday practices whilst their alignment with the rhetoric of informed choice and non-directive care are made present. Once more, Down's syndrome screening is entangled in 'motility' (Latimer 2007; 2013; Latimer and Munro 2006). Here, professionals switch grounds to accomplish screening, in one instance, as a problematic practice – as not very accurate, as opening a can of worms, and as being undertaken routinely and without serious consideration (especially in the case of language barriers) – and in other instances, such as 'frontstage' (Goffman 1959) consultations with parents-to-be, as an acceptable and mostly trouble-free exercise. Here, care is located within abstract medical categories and parents-to-be are figured as exclusively (and morally) responsible for decision-making. This may lead them, accordingly, to self-blame if problems occur for not seriously considering the consequences of undertaking the procedure. This nonalignment with parents-to-be and detachment from, and disposal of, Down's syndrome screening allows professionals, as shown in Chapter 3, to attach themselves to tasks which they invest with value and classify as favoured material for constructing a meaningful work identity. An effect of professionals aligning with the rhetoric of informed choice and non-directive care, then, is creating conditions in which screening – by persisting without possible future complications and professionals' ambiguities coming to the fore – is further routinised in prenatal care.

Sonography and sociality: visualising the unborn

So far in this chapter, I have discussed the downgrading and routinisation of Down's syndrome screening by mostly citing examples from FAD. In SAD, screening is also downgraded by NT scans being refigured from occasions designed to distinguish any possible 'problems' with the foetus or pregnant women into encounters that tender opportunities to meet a 'baby' and reproduce kinship. This argument also extends to ultrasound scans with no association to Down's syndrome screening, namely, dating scans (roughly ten weeks into a pregnancy) and anomaly scans (roughly twenty weeks into a pregnancy). The dating scan and anomaly scan are available in both FAD and SAD. However, they are mostly undertaken in FAD since, as an NHS hospital, each scan is free of charge here. During interviews and in the clinic's backstage (e.g. office chat), professionals regularly accuse parents-to-be, regardless of the ultrasound scan consented to, of not fully comprehending the implications of each respective procedure. In an interview, Rita (FAD midwife) describes her experiences after her recent medical training in dating scans:

> I think women who haven't had a pregnancy before or whose pregnancies have always been fine almost see it as just a chance to see the baby and to find out when the due date is and how many weeks [pregnant] they are. They don't see it as a medical examination to make sure the baby is fine or to see if we can see any problems.

During an interview, Lindsay (FAD midwife) similarly claims:

> Some people are asking you 'can you tell us the sex' [during a dating scan] and I haven't even flipped the monitor around yet to show everything's OK. It's part of the routine. I don't think people really think about what we're doing it for. [...] Women often bring toddlers and

partners too because they see it as a nice scan and as getting a nice picture but it can be problematic if there's no heartbeat or something. But lots of them are quite sensible. They just want to know everything's OK on the scan so a lot of them just come as a two really.

Although Lindsay classifies a range of parents-to-be as 'quite sensible', she says that some parents-to-be do not 'really think about what they're doing [the dating scan] for'. She attributes this to the 'routine' element of ultra-sound, that is, the expectation among parents-to-be that an ultrasound scan is designed to obtain a 'nice picture' of the foetus/baby. According to Lindsay, this becomes problematic, however, when partners and family members attend only to discover the absence of a heartbeat. Similarly, Eve (FAD midwife) establishes a discrepancy between lay and professional knowledge; whilst most women 'come in with half their family' and 'don't know what they're coming to clinic for half the time', professionals are 'more interested in whether [the foetus has] two arms, two legs, and all its anatomy in the right place'. Eve further highlights misconceptions of anomaly scanning since parents-to-be view them solely as encounters to confirm foetal sex. Olivia (SAD sonographer) simi-larly charges parents-to-be with constructing anomaly scans as 'sexing scans', expressing her disapproval that they interpret the procedure as '[having] a little look at the baby'. Francine (FMD head midwife), privy to anomaly scans in her previous role in FAD, claims during an interview that foetal sex is often the first question posed by parents-to-be:

> Very few people appreciate we're looking for abnormalities. Even if you say we're looking for abnormalities, they still don't take it on board. It's reassurance for a lot of people and to get their pictures and to find out the sex of the baby because a lot of women will bring in half the family. The majority of the time this is fine but unfortunately, when you haven't got a good result, it's all the more devastating when it's not normal because you've got your extended family there. That's anomaly scans, NT scans, and dating scans.

Francine claims that anomaly scans are constituted by parents-to-be as opportunities to 'get their pictures and to find out the sex of the baby'. Despite explicit reference to its main purpose, she feels that ultrasound scans are so engrained in the pregnancy imaginary that parents-to-be 'still don't take it on board', opting to invite family members to attend which becomes problematic if a 'good result', translated as the presence of 'normal' markers, is not delivered. Francine's point extends to both anomaly and dating scans together with NT scans for Down's syndrome. Martha (FAD midwife) claims that scans, as 'the glory bits of clinic', are craved by mothers-to-be in particular as they 'are much more interested in having a scan and pictures generally than having anything else'. Fears among professionals about parents-to-be imposing personal interpretations on the function and significance of ultrasound have been reported in earlier research (Draper 2002; Mitchell 2001; Sandelowski 1994a). Ultrasound scans have long been recognised as a 'hybrid practice' (Taylor 1998) with medical and social meanings incorporated into consultations (Roberts 2012), not least in installing an extra monitor for parents-to-be to watch a foetus' movement and the production of 'baby's first picture' (Mitchell 2001). Draper (2002: 787) refers to this as a potential 'clashing of world-views' between the lay paradigm of the ultrasound scan as a social event – in which parents are 'shown' *their* baby (Mitchell and Georges 1997) – and the expert paradigm of it as a medical tool.

In Springtown (and also Freymarsh), whilst professionals' accusations that parents-to-be misinterpret the true intention of ultrasound scans seem valid, they also have an implicit contributory role. In unison with parents-to-be, sonographers in Springtown play their part in configuring the NT scan as a straightforward and entertaining opportunity to meet the baby. This mixing of biomedical purposes with social matters is accomplished in two ways: (1) scans become a 'day out'; (2) scans offer a chance to reproduce kinship. This shows how ultrasound scans are not limited to providing information but also involve sharing meaning in which the logics of 'care', the necessary basis of managing illness or a diagnosis, and 'choice', a concept foregrounded in policy and research where patients are viewed as consumers and active decision-makers, interconnect (Mol 2008). Since my focus is on Down's syndrome screening, I mostly cite extracts taken from SAD observations and interviews with sonographers for the remainder of this chapter.

A day out

The personal and social implications of ultrasound scans have been previously identified. Commentaries on visualising the pregnant-body interior suggest that they offer an opportunity for meeting a 'baby' (Williams et al. 2005), medicalise a pregnancy and erase women in favour of a foetus (Martin 1998), devalue women's knowledge (Sandelowski 1994b), force parents-to-be to tackle moral dilemmas (Gammeltoft 2007), make pregnancies seem more 'real' in the absence of embodied knowledge (Heyman et al. 2006), represent a foetus as a separate and conscious agent (Mitchell and Georges 1997), and prompt appropriate behavioural changes in a partner befitting that of a future parent (Draper 2002). Parents-to-be can experience a range of such conflicting emotions, with enthusiasm and enjoyment often sitting uncomfortably alongside fear and anxiety during a scan (Williams et al. 2005). In short, ultrasound imaging allows parents to reflect on, and rework, their experiences of pregnancy by providing a way of knowing and feeling the foetus through the coupling of human and machine (Mitchell 2001; Mitchell and Georges 1997).

In Freymarsh and Springtown, ultrasound scans are constructed as important and meaningful events for visualising a foetus. Take, for example, the following fieldnotes from an echocardiography scan carried out by Dr Torres (FMD cardiologist) in which there is a suspicion of a foetal heart defect:

> Dr Torres, Jodi (FMD cardiac physiologist), Mr and Mrs O'Neill (parents-to-be), and their three daughters (Cassie, Nina, and Sian) are in the scan room. Dr Torres begins and, after a few minutes of scanning, turns to the children:

> DR TORRES: Now you have to pay me for this show [Mr and Mrs O'Neill, Cassie, Nina, and Sian laugh]. And if you can't pay, you'll have to do your mum's chores. You'll have to do the washing, cook the food, and massage her feet.
> MRS O'NEILL: Not my feet, they wouldn't want to go anywhere near them!

> During the scan, Dr Torres utters 'it looks good so far', 'it all looks fine', 'there's nothing abnormal here', and 'there's nothing to be concerned about':

> DR TORRES: [Pointing to Cassie, Nina, and Sian] Do you see the head and the brain there, girls?
> CASSIE: Is that the brain [points]?
> DR TORRES: That is the brain. There's the head, the brain, two little legs trying to kick mummy [all laugh].
> JODI: Baby's legs are all stretched out there!
> DR TORRES: I'm just trying to get a good profile. The girls came here for a show and mum has come here for a show, so let's give them a day out! You have a shy baby here, like you girls I think [turns to Cassie, Nina, and Sian].

> Dr Torres scans for another few seconds:

> DR TORRES: I think we can stop the scan there. Everything is fine though.
> MRS O'NEILL: I'm so relieved. Thank you so much.
> MR O'NEILL: Brilliant. Thanks doctor.

Following the suspicion of a heart defect being disproved, Dr Torres describes how the daughters must 'pay a fee for the show', how failure to pay will result in 'doing your mum's chores', and how the foetus is 'shy' and 'trying to kick mommy'. Whilst Dr Torres' playfulness can be attributed to an attempt to relax the O'Neill's following a suspected defect (Dr Torres also reassures the O'Neill's with utterances such as 'it looks good so far' and 'there's nothing abnormal here'), it additionally points to how ultrasound scans, used principally for detecting potential problems with a foetus or pregnant woman, can be refigured as what Dr Torres calls 'a day out'. Later in the day, Dr Torres is explaining a suspected large inlet ventricular septal defect[4] and dextro-transposition of the great arteries[5] to Mr and Mrs Hall (parents-to-be). After explaining that the situation 'is incredibly rare and most cardiac specialists don't even have a clue about this', Dr Torres draws a picture of the heart and associated defect to explain the situation.

Here, materials are produced and used in the production of care, with ultrasound scans and, on occasions, sketches (e.g. of cardiac defects) becoming physical resources of knowledge and reassurance. In the absence of a suspected defect, however, an ultrasound scan can be constructed as a day out, an entertaining and enjoyable excursion where parents-to-be interact with *their* baby. In SAD, the NT scan is often afforded such a reconstruction. The following fieldnotes are taken from the opening exchanges of an NT scan between Olivia (SAD sonographer), Mr and Mrs Fox (parents-to-be), and Mrs Fox's mother:

> OLIVIA: Baby's trying to stand up by the looks of things! Do you see the hand?
> MRS FOX: Yes!
> MOTHER: Ah look at that. The heart looks like it's going well.
> OLIVIA: Yes it is.
> MRS FOX: Ah I can see it moving!
> OLIVIA: Baby's having a little wriggle.
> MRS FOX: Look at the arms there!
> MOTHER: He's doing the Usain Bolt [celebration]!
> MR FOX: Flipping heck, this is amazing.
> OLIVIA: Seeing is believing isn't it?
> MRS FOX: You don't think it's real until you see it like this.
> MR FOX: It probably just feels like you've eaten too much curry! [all laugh].
> MRS FOX: It definitely makes it more real. [...] Is that a hand there?
> OLIVIA: Yes.
> MRS FOX: Wow. I didn't know you could see so much at this stage.
> OLIVIA: Baby's having a little dance in there now!
> MR FOX: Having a bit of fun!
> OLIVIA: Do you see the arms moving? Baby looks like it's doing backstroke.
> MR AND MRS FOX: Yes [laugh]!
> OLIVIA: And the head there too. There's the nasal bone [points]. That's a good sign that it's there because if it's absent, that can be a sign of a problem.
> MRS FOX: OK.
> OLIVIA: So what we're looking at today is the nuchal fold which is the fluid which collects at the back of your baby's neck.

Olivia explains the NT scan, its outcomes, and the implications of such outcomes. Measurements are taken at an average of 1.06mm. Olivia explains a measurement under 3mm is 'good'.

The upsurge of visualisation technologies in medicine relies on professionals who must make imaging meaningful for everyone involved. With parents-to-be, sonographers like Olivia engage in 'collaborative coding' (Roberts 2012: 299), fashioning meanings out of signs and symbols forged in conjunction with one another. Mr and Mrs Fox – in accord with Olivia and Mrs Fox's mother – describe the baby as 'having a little wriggle', as 'having a little dance', as 'having a bit of fun', and as 'doing the Usain Bolt [celebration]'. They also identify anatomical landmarks (e.g. 'look at the arms', 'is that a hand?'). Mr Fox describes the NT scan as 'amazing', with his partner suggesting the pregnancy does not seem real 'until you see it like this'. Olivia finally draws attention to the primary purpose of the scan with reference to the nasal bone, its presence reducing the prospect of a 'problem' being found in the foetus.

As highlighted above, there is frequently a large degree of humour and informality during NT scans. The casualness is perpetuated further via chit-chat during scans, such as professionals asking parents-to-be about plans for the weekend and how many other children parents-to-be have (or are planning to have). Whilst this informality and joviality occasionally emerges in screening consultations at FAD, this increases in SAD on receipt of a visual representation of a foetus at play on a large television monitor (not available at FAD). In the extract described above, Olivia and Mr and Mrs Fox prioritise the entertaining component of an ultrasound scan over establishing the purpose of this procedure. Such playful encounters may be harmless and designed to alleviate the angst of, and offer reassurance to, parents-to-be. But they also help reconstruct the NT scan as a 'day out'. This reflects how parents-to-be occasionally claim that they are unaware of the purpose of the procedure being undertaken. During an NT scan, for instance, Mrs Jackson (mother-to-be) is accompanied by her sister and mother and claims she 'does not know anything' about the procedure. After Sophie (SAD sonographer) describes the scan, Mrs Jackson's sister video-records the imaging displayed on the monitor and, once measurements are defined by Sophie as 'nice and small', Mrs Jackson seems rather uninterested in this information and enquires as to foetal sex (Sophie says that she cannot determine this at the current stage of gestation).

The pursuit of acquiring a material memory of the baby (not 'foetus', as ultrasound helps *make* the baby) and unmasking its sex, together with the presence of family members, highlights how scans can mostly become a day out rather than ensuring – drawing on Eve's earlier contentions – 'whether [the foetus has] two arms, two legs, and all its anatomy in the right place'. During NT scans, parents-to-be (or one mother-to-be) can sometimes be accompanied by friends. The following fieldnotes are taken from an NT scan with Esther (SAD sonographer), Mrs Fowler (mother-to-be), and two of Mrs Fowler's friends:

ESTHER: Do you know much about the NT scan?
MRS FOWLER: No, not really.

ESTHER: Do you know it's a screening test for Down's syndrome?

MRS FOWLER: Yes.

ESTHER: Well this screening test gives you a risk of having a baby with Down's syndrome. It measures a pad of fluid which collects at the back of the baby's neck. It appears between ten and fourteen weeks and disappears after fourteen weeks but we're still not quite sure why. But when it's enlarged, it's associated with chromosomal abnormalities.

MRS FOWLER: Is it just Down's syndrome?

ESTHER: No. It also looks for two other chromosomal abnormalities. Your bloods are taken and these are combined with the size of the baby, your age, and the NT which is calculated into a risk factor. This gives you a risk factor for Down's syndrome, Edward's syndrome, and Patau syndrome. We can't screen for all abnormalities so we test for three of the most common, two of the most lethal. We like the NT under three millimetres and we need baby to be still so we can measure it. The good thing about this test as well is the false positive rate is lower.[6] That's one of the benefits you get of having the scan done earlier. You'll get the results on Thursday. Our cut-off here for a high-risk and a low-risk is 1 in 150. So if you get lower than 1 in 150, you'll get a higher-risk result and you'll be advised to have an amniocentesis. Baby gets a gold star because it's been the best behaved we've had tonight [Mrs Fowler and friends laugh].

MRS FOWLER: Good!

ESTHER: Baby's using your cervix as a bouncy castle there!

MRS FOWLER: I can see!

ESTHER: There are the eyes, nose, the Buddha belly [Mrs Fowler and friends laugh], arms, bum, legs, back of the head too. We check the back of the head to look for other abnormalities too.

MRS FOWLER: But is everything looking OK?

ESTHER: Everything is looking normal. The NT is nice and small. Oh look, there's two legs there!

After Mrs Fowler conveys her lack of knowledge about screening, Esther provides an explanation. After fulfilling her duties of providing medically correct information as part of the governing principles of non-directive care and informed choice, Esther quips that 'baby gets a gold star because it's the best behaved we've had tonight'. Esther subsequently claims that the baby is using Mrs Fowler's cervix 'as a bouncy castle' before making the imaging on the monitor meaningful for Mrs Fowler and her guests by establishing anatomical features such as the eyes, nose, and 'Buddha belly'.

Throughout NT scans, sonographers and parents-to-be identify physical features or movements of the baby and ascribe these to personality traits ('what a poser', 'you've got a stubborn one', 'baby is well-behaved tonight', 'it's a very photogenic baby', 'cheeky baby just flicked us the finger!', 'you've got a very chilled out baby'; 'the muppet won't behave, that little joker!'; 'the baby's been very active so can you check it's not a frog instead of a baby!?'), a favourable physical appearance ('what a cutie', 'our baby's beautiful', 'you've got such a little doll there', 'so pretty', 'beautiful'), and certain activities such as dancing ('baby's doing a little jig', 'you've got a baby Michael Flatley in there', 'baby's doing a bit of ballet') and playing sports ('you've got a rugby player in there', 'baby's going to be a footballer with a kick like that', 'we've got a future gymnast'). The description of a foetus as a rugby player or gymnast through such 'belly talk' (Han 2013) often corresponds to hetero-normative gender ideals. During an NT scan, hetero-normative gender roles and expectations are often erected, even before foetal sex is determined (perhaps implicitly revealing, thus, the preferences of parents-to-be). Nonetheless, the ascription of personality traits, expectations, and conduct in the baby – alongside the presence of family and friends during NT scans – frames the procedure as an enjoyable expedition as opposed to, in Rita's (FAD midwife) words, a 'medical examination'.

Reproducing kinship

Ultrasound scans in Springtown, and particularly NT scans, are frequently attended by parents-to-be and other family members (most likely to be children). The attendance of children may be circumstantial, rather than being an active choice, such as being unable to arrange childcare. However, children often still attend the procedure along with fathers-to-be (or same-sex partners, but mostly fathers-to-be). In FAD, fathers-to-be and children – if present at all – regularly remain in the waiting room whilst mothers-to-be are invited for a consultation. In contrast, at SAD, they regularly attend screening consultations. Their presence in NT scans undoubtedly stems from the visualisation of a foetus and the scans being refigured as events in which parents-to-be – and others – welcome a new family member. Accounting for his and his wife's presence during an NT scan, for instance, Maurice (grandfather) claims that his attendance can be attributed to '[wanting] to come along today to meet our latest grandchild'. The following fieldnotes are taken from an NT scan between Olivia (SAD sonographer) and Mr and Mrs Carlisle (parents-to-be):

> OLIVIA: Baby's swimming! There's the arm stretched right above the head, the stomach, and the leg [pointing].
> MR CARLISLE: Wow.
> MRS CARLISLE: Ah. This is much better than the last scan. We got such a terrible picture last time!
> MR CARLISLE: That is amazing.
> OLIVIA: So we're looking at the NT here. Do you see these white lines and the black fluid in-between [points]? That's the NT and I can see

it is tiny. We want it under three millimetres and it definitely is. Now are you going to turn over and give mum a good picture?

MRS CARLISLE: He's being shy!

OLIVIA: Baby's being difficult! I'll try and coerce baby into moving. Which way are you going to go, baby?

MR CARLISLE: The baby must be like me. Never listens!

MRS CARLISLE: He's got that from you! [Olivia takes measurements of the NT as around 1.67mm].

OLIVIA: Lovely, fantastic, that's miles under. Are you going to roll over, baby?

MR CARLISLE: He doesn't want to play at all does he?

MRS CARLISLE: He's going 'get off! Who the hell is that?'

MR CARLISLE: He's stubborn.

OLIVIA: Yes, it definitely is a boy! [All laugh] Baby is being very naughty now.

MR CARLISLE: Come on! I think he's moving. Or she.

MRS CARLISLE: It's definitely a boy. He's just like his Dad!

OLIVIA: He's being very lazy. You can sleep all night, can't you baby?! I want to get a picture. Come on stop teasing! Baby's a little rascal.

After a few seconds, the baby's face appears on the monitor. This is met with cheers from Olivia and Mr and Mrs Carlisle. Some pictures are taken and handed to Mr Carlisle.

Throughout much of the scan, Mr and Mrs Carlisle engage in what Kroløkke (2011: 26) defines as 'ultra-gasms', namely utterances or 'response cries' (Goffman 1981) conveying a sense of awe or amazement at the imaging on the monitor ('*wow*', '*ah*'). This seems to challenge popular claims, particularly in feminist literature, that ultrasound erases women in favour of the foetus. Here, and in other scans, parents-to-be are active participants, not disembodied onlookers, in co-creating the baby and identifying some maternal features. Prior to soliciting any information regarding the screening procedure, Mrs Carlisle praises the clarity of imaging in contrast to the 'terrible picture' received following a previous scan. After establishing a seemingly small NT, Olivia urges the baby to 'turn over' and 'give mum a good picture'. Mrs Carlisle associates movement to 'being shy', referring to the baby as a 'he' throughout much of the consultation in the absence of knowledge regarding the baby's sex. Mr Carlisle playfully associates the lack of movement to his own personality characteristics ('he must be like me. Never listens!'), before Mrs Carlisle confirms 'he's got that from you!'

In the consultation between Olivia and Mr and Mrs Carlisle, the focus appears to be on creating pictures, ascribing gender expectations, and on reproducing family via 'resemblance talk' (Becker et al. 2005: 1300). Morgan (1996) identifies family relationships as processes that are fluid, complex, and variable. Kinship is symbolic rather than being 'natural' or biologically driven

(Franklin 1997; Strathern 1992), yet great significance is attached to genetic or blood relationships. Such 'family practices' (Morgan 1996) emerge in the ultrasound room, particularly with the creation of an ultrasound image, that is, a material souvenir for parents-to-be and family members to take home. Sonographers construct the imaging on screen *into* a baby by drawing on visible markers of personhood and familial resemblances, thereby 'weaving the foetus into a network of kinship relations' (Mitchell 2001: 134). Familial exchanges are encouraged via the identification of anatomical features replicating either or both parents-to-be. In one example, Esther points out the 'nasal bone' to which Mr Dalton replies 'I hope the baby has got [Mrs Dalton's] nose!' Esther laughs but responds that 'the nasal bone being absent can have problems linked with Down's syndrome so it's good it's there'. Whilst Esther attaches to the medical dimension of ultrasound scanning, Mr Dalton opts for a nonmedical interpretation. For the most part, however, professionals participate in constructing screening as an opportunity to meet a baby. This, in effect, contributes to trivialising it as a routine and taken-for-granted practice.

'A very different atmosphere'

I have outlined midwives' and sonographers' accounts which identify the problems caused by parents-to-be, allegedly, treating ultrasound as a social event and, as such, not fully comprehending the implications of this practice. For instance, Esther (SAD sonographer) claims that parents-to-be do not realise the true purpose of ultrasound and, subsequently, do them 'willy-nilly'. If midwives and sonographers express such concerns, why do they do this work and why do they persist in promoting a jovial, informal atmosphere? If parents-to-be expect the primary output of NT scans to be the acquisition of 'pretty pictures' (Lisa, SAD sonographer), why are they not scrapped? During an interview, Sophie (SAD sonographer) describes her approach when performing NT scans:

> People do have ultrasound scans just for fun. Personally, I always try and check everything's OK first because it's a very different atmosphere in the room if you've got a nuchal fold measuring 4.0mm to one that's measuring 1.2mm and you've got a baby lying there kicking its legs and waving because a nice small nuchal translucency is very good news on a scan. I know we've got to check all other factors but if it's good news and it's positive, as long as everything's OK, I usually am quite relaxed and chat with people as that's what they want. They do want a first scan, they want nice pictures, and they want the baby waving.

Sophie suggests that the perceived absence of any serious concern ('[a nuchal translucency] measuring 1.2mm') allows her to create an appropriate atmosphere in which a baby is not only announced when there is 'very good news' but is also coded according to movements ('a baby lying there kicking its legs and waving) and validated by producing material memories ('they do want a first scan, they want nice pictures, and they want the baby waving'). Sophie, however, claims that the absence of 'good news' would create 'a very different atmosphere', intimating that she would not produce 'waving' images of the baby should a problem be suspected. I observed only one NT scan where a problem was suspected. Esther (sonographer) told Mr and Mrs Tomkins (parents-to-be) that she believed the foetus had cystic hygroma[7] which she explained is linked to Turner syndrome. Much like Sophie intimates, the scan took on a 'very different atmosphere' in which playful exchanges, regularly a staple of the ultrasound encounter, became absent.

Interestingly, even when the foetus was (temporally) classified as 'normal', the atmosphere was not always jovial and informal in NT scans. The following fieldnotes are taken from an NT scan between Esther (SAD sonographer) and Mr and Mrs Williams (parents-to-be):

MRS WILLIAMS: I'm a bit nervous because we're IVF.[8]
ESTHER: OK. Let's have a look. Do you see this black gap between these two white lines? That's the NT. When it's enlarged, it's associated with chromosomal abnormalities. We want the NT below three millimetres. [Esther continues to describe the procedure] There's the little Buddha belly there!
MRS WILLIAMS: Like mine then [smiles].
ESTHER: Now let's look at that NT.
MR WILLIAMS: It's that bottom black line, is it?
ESTHER: Yes. It's this line here to this line here [pointing]. We take three measurements and usually take the largest of them all.
MRS WILLIAMS: It's quite scary isn't it?
MR WILLIAMS: Just relax.
ESTHER: Yes just relax. Where are you going to deliver?
MRS WILLIAMS: Watermont. Is this OK?
ESTHER: Of course!
MRS WILLIAMS: We're consultant-led care as well. Does the baby have enough room in there?
ESTHER: Yes, baby's got plenty of room. And baby looks to have the hiccups now!
MRS WILLIAMS: But he definitely has enough room?
ESTHER: Yes. That's just me pressing down with the transducer so don't worry.
MR WILLIAMS: So on looking initially, it's the size of [pause].
ESTHER: Small. It's a small size which is good.
MRS WILLIAMS: Good.
MR WILLIAMS: Great.

During the scan, Mrs Williams becomes 'nervous' and 'scared' owing to her IVF treatment. Several parents-to-be are anxious prior to a scan and, admittedly, do not necessarily subscribe to constructing the procedure as an enjoyable excursion. This worry was most common in mothers-to-be over the age of thirty-five who, with a 'higher-risk' of having a foetus with Down's syndrome, frequently accounted for their decision to have screening by citing their age. When parents-to-be had previous pregnancy complications or other concerns, sonographers – explicitly or implicitly – adjusted their body language and interpretation of the imaging. They toned down the enjoyable component of NT scans and prioritised medical information ahead of its personal, social meanings. This is reflected in Dr Karman (FMD consultant) only undertaking NT scans, albeit on a rare occasion, with parents-to-be who have current, or had previous, pregnancy complications including recurrent miscarriages or a history of chromosomal conditions. Otherwise, Dr Karman is granted immunity from, to return to an earlier sentiment, the *easy stuff* which *clogs up the clinic*. Thus, NT scans are expected to proceed without a setback by producing a lower-risk result.

However, whilst not all screening consultations in Springtown are reconstructed as enjoyable days out and opportunities to welcome new family members, this is a common situation. The boundaries between the medical and social components of a scan are often shifting, permeable, and difficult to untangle (Roberts 2012). In SAD, this can be linked to sonographers working in a privately funded setting. In Springtown, care is overtly organised, more than NHS hospitals, around an ethos of individual consumption where professionals tailor treatment in line with a recognisable cultural script (Kerr 2013; Strong 1979). This is problematic for professionals who must negotiate the tension between medical care and consumer choice, that is, they must balance authentic/entertaining experiences (e.g. small talk, laughing, identifying positive attributes of the baby, drawing smiley faces on the abdomen with ultrasound gel) with clinical expertise to reassure and pacify parents-to-be.

Owing to the commoditisation of their practice, sonographers must engage in two forms of 'emotional labour' (Hochschild 1983). First, they work hard to reassure parents-to-be and repair potentially fractured encounters via interactional exchanges emphasising the baby's 'normality' or favourable features as well as the apparent rarity of medical 'problems'. Second, sonographers must also put on a show. Skilfully and enthusiastically involving parents-to-be whilst erecting a lively, homely, and pleasant atmosphere is encouraged in a situation where silence may indicate a prospective problem (Thomas 2015). What is suggested here, then, is that their imperative to merge medical information with a consumer-friendly performance indirectly, and I assume unintentionally, trivialises Down's syndrome screening and downgrades its value as a medical procedure; it becomes, once again, something done as a matter of routine.

Summary

I began this chapter by identifying the tensions between the accounts and practices of professionals. In their accounts, professionals identify their own alignment with the rhetoric of informed choice and non-directive care. However, they also have concerns and anxieties about Down's syndrome screening, such as its inaccuracy and its capacity to 'open a can of worms'. In practice, professionals draw upon this discursive resource of informed choice and non-directive care to shape their approach. During consultations with parents-to-be, they bestow them with a glut of information and, in essence, leave the decision up to them. Bosk (1992: 10) refers to this classification of choice as grounds for accomplishing 'patient abandonment' whereby the satisfaction of a professional's care obligation is not taking charge of decision-making, that is, acting but not acting decisively. Although I avoid the term abandonment, I similarly show that in Freymarsh and Springtown, policies of informed choice and non-directive care – enacted by professionals who must communicate neutral scientific representations to parents-to-be in screening consultations – are mobilised to locate (moral) responsibility for screening in the hands of parents-to-be and to prevent professionals from becoming entangled with problematic concerns (Strange 2015). With parents-to-be enacted as rational and logical choice-makers, screening is constituted as a matter of personal rather than professional concern (Latimer 2000), despite professionals playing an active role in shaping this practice.

However, parents-to-be are often described as not being attuned to the seriousness of Down's syndrome screening and, so, as submissively opting for the procedure. This trend has been recorded in this fieldwork and in the literature, with parents-to-be seemingly consenting to Down's syndrome screening as an instance of conformity rather than being the product of any active decision-making processes (Heyman et al. 2006; Lippman 1994; Marteau 1995; Santalahti et al. 1998; Tsouroufli 2011). Choices are far from free, with the divide between voluntary choice and socially enforced coercion being blurred (Kerr et al. 1998). Combined with professionals' disposal of screening, and their personal concerns about the practice being curbed on the premise of assuring informed choice/non-directive care, this creates conditions in which Down's syndrome screening is accomplished as an expected moment in pregnancy rituals. With no critical engagement from either professionals or parents-to-be, it remains a taken-for-granted and unquestioned component of prenatal care.

In the second part of this chapter, I revealed how ultrasound scans are constructed as enjoyable 'days out' where parents-to-be and family members meet their 'baby' and reconstruct kinship, thereby undermining ultrasound as an occasion where any medical concerns with a foetus or pregnant woman are identified. This accomplishes two things. First, Down's syndrome screening is refigured as a routine part of prenatal care. The rituals of opting for ultrasound, obtaining pictures, and inviting family and friends to the scan – as well as recreating family narratives – accomplish a disengagement with the technology's main function. Alongside professionals' obligation to merge medical information with consumer-friendly performances, this trivialises Down's syndrome screening and downgrades its value as a medical procedure.

Second, Down's syndrome screening – by becoming constructed as a day out and particularly as a chance for reproducing kinship – accomplishes the production of ideal/expected bodies and future families in relation to both biological kinship and wider cultural values. During ultrasound, the playful exchanges as described above pass through a 'cultural sieve' whereby professionals select the best and most reassuring features to highlight (Mitchell and Georges 1997; Thomas 2015). The ascription of physical features and movements of the baby to personality traits, favourable physical appearances, and gendered conduct configures certain ideals of bodies that become normatively expected but that are often based on problematic cultural ideologies. This shapes bodies and families in ways that may not correlate with future outcomes, such as a diagnosis of disability. This is reflected in NT scans becoming either 'days out' or encounters that take on 'a very different atmosphere'. Whilst the former reinforce ideas of a 'normal' body, the latter strengthen the category of an 'abnormal' or 'potentially abnormal' body. Chapters 5 and 6 extend this focus by attending to how Down's syndrome itself is classified, or not, within prenatal care (Chapter 5) and how this connects with notions of normality and perfection in this setting (Chapter 6).

Notes

1   The evidence for this is not provided in this extract. However, it seems to reflect claims elsewhere that only around 1 in 20 to 1 in 30 screen-positive results correctly identify an affected pregnancy (Buckley and Buckley 2008). Buckley and Buckley say that this encourages many mothers-to-be with unaffected pregnancies to accept an invasive diagnostic procedure (amniocentesis/CVS) that, in some cases, leads to a miscarriage.

2   After an amniocentesis, a sample of amniotic fluid is sent to a cytogenetics lab for chromosome analysis. This potentially leads to the detection of conditions including, but not limited to, Down's syndrome, Edward's syndrome, Patau syndrome, cystic fibrosis, muscular dystrophy, sickle-cell disease, neural tube defects (spina bifida and anencephaly), and Tay Sachs disease.

3   Emma is also an FMD midwife but I observed her most frequently in FAD.

4   An inlet ventricular septal defect is a hole in the septum near where the blood enters the ventricles through the tricuspid and mitral valves.

5   Dextro-transposition of the great arteries is a cardiac defect in which the two main arteries carrying the blood out of the heart – the main pulmonary artery and the aorta – are switched in position.

6   In screening, a false-positive means that a mother-to-be receives a positive result but the foetus does not have a diagnosis of Down's syndrome.

7   Cystic hygromas are abnormal growths, often developing in the womb, that usually appear on the head or neck of a foetus.

8 IVF (in-vitro fertilisation) is a process by which an egg cell is fertilised by sperm outside of the body. It is a major treatment for infertility once other methods of assisted reproductive technology have failed.

Bibliography

Ahmed, S., Bryant, L.D. and Cole, P. 2013. Midwives' perceptions of their role as facilitators of informed choice in antenatal screening. *Midwifery* 29(7), pp. 745–750.
Allen, D. 2013. 'Just a typical teenager': the social ecology of 'normal adolescence' – insights from diabetes care. *Symbolic Interaction* 36(1), pp. 40–59.
Aune, I. and Möller, A. 2012. 'I want choice, but I don't want to decide': a qualitative study of pregnant women's experiences regarding early ultrasound risk assessment for chromosomal anomalies. *Midwifery* 28(1), pp. 14–23.
Becker, G., Butler, A. and Nachtigall, R.D. 2005. Resemblance talk: a challenge for parents whose children were conceived with donor gametes in the US. *Social Science and Medicine* 61(6), pp. 1300–1309.
Berg, M. 1992. The construction of medical disposals: medical sociology and medical problem solving in clinical practice. *Sociology of Health and Illness* 14(2), pp. 151–180.
Bosk, C.L. 1992. *All God's Mistakes: Genetic Counseling in a Pediatric Hospital*. Chicago: University of Chicago Press.
Browner, C.H., Preloran, H.M. and Press, N. 1996. The effects of ethnicity, education and an informational video on pregnant women's knowledge and decisions about a prenatal diagnostic screening test. *Patient Education and Counselling* 27(2), pp. 135–146.
Buckley, F. and Buckley, S.J. 2008. Wrongful deaths and rightful lives: screening for Down syndrome. *Down Syndrome Research and Practice* 12(2), pp. 79–86.
Burton-Jeangros, C., Cavalli, S., Gouilhers, S. and Hammer, R. 2013. Between tolerable uncertainty and unacceptable risks: how health professionals and pregnant women think about the probabilities generated by prenatal screening. *Health, Risk and Society* 15(2), pp. 144–161.
Clarke, A. 1991. Is non-directive genetic counselling possible? *Lancet* 338(8773), pp. 998–1001.
Cunningham-Burley, S. and Kerr, A. 1999. Defining the 'social': towards an understanding of scientific and medical discourses on the social aspects of the new human genetics. *Sociology of Health and Illness* 21(5), pp. 647–668.
Draper, J. 2002. 'It was a real good show': the ultrasound scan, fathers and the power of visual knowledge. *Sociology of Health and Illness* 24(6), pp. 771–795.
Foucault, M. 1973. *The Birth of the Clinic: An Archaeology of Medical Perception*. London: Tavistock Publications.
Franklin, S. 1997. *Embodied Progress: A Cultural Account of Assisted Conception*. New York: Routledge.
Gammeltoft, T.M. 2007. Prenatal diagnosis in postwar Vietnam: power, subjectivity, and citizenship. *American Anthropologist* 109(1), pp. 153–163.
Garfinkel, H. 1967. *Studies in Ethnomethodology*. Englewood Cliffs, NJ: Prentice-Hall.
Goffman, E. 1959. *The Presentation of Self in Everyday Life*. London: Allen Lane.
Goffman, E. 1981. *Forms of Talk*. Philadelphia: University of Pennsylvania Press.
Green, J.M. and Statham, H. 1996. Psychosocial aspects of prenatal screening and diagnosis. In: Marteau, T.M. and Richards, M. eds. *The Troubled Helix: Social and*

Psychological Implications of the New Human Genetics. New York: Cambridge University Press, pp. 140–163.

Han, S. 2013. *Pregnancy in Practice: Expectation and Experience in the Contemporary US*. Oxford: Berghahn Books.

Hey, M. and Hurst, K. 2003. Antenatal screening: why do women refuse? *RCM Midwives Journal* 6(5), pp. 216–220.

Heyman, B., Hundy, G., Sandall, J., Spencer, K., Williams, C., Grellier, R. and Pitson, L. 2006. On being at higher risk: a qualitative study of prenatal screening for chromosomal anomalies. *Social Science and Medicine* 62(10), pp. 2360–2372.

Hochschild, A. 1983. *The Managed Heart: Commercialization of Human Feeling*. Berkeley: University of California Press.

Hunt, L., de Voogd, K.B. and Castañeda, H. 2005. The routine and the traumatic in prenatal genetic diagnosis: does clinical information inform patient decision-making? *Patient Education and Counselling* 56(3), pp. 302–312.

Ivry, T. 2006. At the backstage of prenatal care: Japanese ob-gyns negotiating prenatal diagnosis. *Medical Anthropology Quarterly* 20(4), pp. 441–468.

Kerr, A. 2013. Body work in assisted conception: exploring public and private settings. *Sociology of Health and Illness* 35(3), pp. 465–478.

Kerr, A. and Cunningham-Burley, S. 2000. On ambivalence and risk: reflexive modernity and the new human genetics. *Sociology* 43(2), pp. 283–304.

Kerr, A., Cunningham-Burley, S. and Amos, A. 1998. Eugenics and the new genetics in Britain: examining contemporary professionals' accounts. *Science, Technology and Human Values* 23(2), 175–198.

Krøløkke, C. 2011. Biotourist performances: doing parenting during the ultrasound. *Text and Performance Quarterly* 31(1), pp. 15–36.

Latimer, J.E. 1997. Giving patients a future: the constituting of classes in an acute medical unit. *Sociology of Health and Illness* 19(2), pp. 160–185.

Latimer, J.E. 2000. *The Conduct of Care: Understanding Nursing Practice*. Oxford: Blackwell Science.

Latimer, J.E. 2007. Diagnosis, dysmorphology, and the family: knowledge, motility, choice. *Medical Anthropology* 26(2), pp. 97–138.

Latimer, J.E. 2013. *The Gene, the Clinic and the Family: Diagnosing Dysmorphology, Reviving Medical Dominance*. London: Routledge.

Latimer, J.E. and Munro, R. 2006. Driving the social. *The Sociological Review* 54(SI), pp. 32–53.

Lippman, A. 1994. The genetic construction of prenatal testing: choice, consent, or conformity for women? In: Rothenberg, K. and Thomson, E. eds. *Women and Prenatal Testing: Facing the Challenges of Genetic Technology*. Columbus: Ohio State University Press, pp. 9–34.

Markens, S., Browner, C.H. and Press, N. 1999. 'Because of the risks': how US pregnant women account for refusing prenatal screening. *Social Science and Medicine* 49(3), pp. 359–369.

Marteau, T.M. 1995. Towards informed decisions about prenatal testing: a review. *Prenatal Diagnosis* 15(13), pp. 1215–1226.

Martin, E. 1998. The fetus as intruder: mother's bodies and medical metaphors. In: Davis-Floyd, R.E. and Dumit, J. eds. *Cyborg Babies: From Techo-Sex to Techno-Tots*. New York: Routledge, pp. 125–142.

Mitchell, L.M. 2001. *Baby's First Picture: Ultrasound and the Politics of Fetal Subjects*. Toronto: University of Toronto Press.

Mitchell, L.M. and Georges, E. 1997. Cross-cultural cyborgs: Greek and Canadian women's discourses on fetal ultrasound. *Feminist Studies* 23(2), pp. 373–401.

Mol, A.M. 2002. *The Body Multiple: Ontology in Medical Practice*. Durham, NC: Duke University Press.

Mol, A.M. 2008. *The Logic of Care: Health and the Problem of Patient Choice*. New York: Routledge.

Mol, A.M. and Law, J. 2004. Embodied action, enacted bodies: the example of hypoglycaemia. *Body and Society* 10(2–3), pp. 43–62.

Morgan, D.H.G. 1996. *Family Connections: An Introduction to Family Studies*. Cambridge: Polity Press.

Pilnick, A. 2008. 'It's something for you both to think about': choice and decision-making in nuchal translucency screening for Down's syndrome. *Sociology of Health and Illness* 30(4), pp. 511–530.

Pilnick, A., Fraser, D.M. and James, D.K. 2004. Presenting and discussing nuchal translucency screening for fetal abnormality in the UK. *Midwifery* 20(1), pp. 82–93.

Pilnick, A. and Zayts, O. 2012. 'Let's have it tested first': choice and circumstances in decision-making following positive antenatal screening in Hong Kong. *Sociology of Health and Illness* 34(2), pp. 266–282.

Rapp, R. 2000. *Testing Women, Testing the Fetus: The Social Impact of Amniocentesis in America*. London: Routledge.

Remennick, L. 2006. The quest for the perfect baby: why do Israeli women seek prenatal genetic testing? *Sociology of Health and Illness* 28(1), pp. 21–53.

Roberts, J. 2012. 'Wakey wakey baby': narrating four-dimensional (4D) bonding scans. *Sociology of Health and Illness* 34(2), pp. 299–314.

Sandelowski, M. 1994a. Channel of desire: fetal ultrasonography in two use-contexts. *Qualitative Health Research* 4(3), pp. 262–280.

Sandelowski, M. 1994b. Separate, but less unequal: fetal ultrasonography and the transformation of expectant mother/fatherhood. *Gender and Society* 8(2), pp. 230–245.

Santalahti, P., Hemminki, E., Latikka, A.M. and Ryynanen, M. 1998. Women's decision making in prenatal screening. *Social Science and Medicine* 46(8), pp. 1067–1076.

Schwennesen, N. and Koch, L. 2012. Representing and intervening: 'doing' good care in first trimester prenatal knowledge production and decision-making. *Sociology of Health and Illness* 34(2), pp. 282–298.

Scott, S., Hinton-Smith, T., Härmä, V. and Broome, K. 2013. Goffman in the gallery: interactive art and visitor shyness. *Symbolic Interaction* 36(4), pp. 417–438.

Shakespeare, T.W. 2011. Choices, reasons and feelings: prenatal diagnosis as disability dilemma. *European Journal of Disability Research* 5(1), pp. 37–43.

Silverman, D. 1987. *Communication and Medical Practice: Social Relations in the Clinic*. London: Sage.

Strange, H. 2015. *Non-invasive Prenatal Diagnosis: The Emergence and Translation of a New Prenatal Testing Technology*. Unpublished Ph.D. Thesis, Cardiff University.

Strathern, M. 1992. *Reproducing the Future: Anthropology, Kinship, and the New Reproductive Technologies*. New York: Routledge.

Strong, P. 1979. *The Ceremonial Order of the Clinic: Parents, Doctors and Medical Bureaucracies*. Henley-on-Thames: Routledge and Kegan Paul.

Taylor, J.S. 1998. Image of contradiction: obstetrical ultrasound in American culture. In: Franklin, S. and Ragoné, H. eds. *Reproducing Reproduction: Kinship, Power and Technological Innovation*. Philadelphia: University of Pennsylvania Press, pp. 15–45.

Thomas, G.M. 2015. Picture perfect: '4D' ultrasound and the commoditisation of the private prenatal clinic. *Journal of Consumer Culture* [Online first].

Tsouroufli, M. 2011. Routinisation and constraints on informed choice in a one-stop clinic offering first trimester chromosomal antenatal screening for Down's syndrome. *Midwifery* 27(4), pp. 431–436.

Williams, C., Alderson, P. and Farsides, B. 2002a. Dilemmas encountered by health practitioners offering nuchal translucency screening: a qualitative case study. *Prenatal Diagnosis* 22(3), pp. 216–220.

Williams, C., Alderson, P. and Farsides, B. 2002b. Is nondirectiveness possible within the context of antenatal screening and testing? *Social Science and Medicine* 54(3), pp. 339–347.

Williams, C., Sandall, J., Lewando-Hundt, G., Heyman, B., Spencer, K. and Grellier, R. 2005. Women as moral pioneers? Experiences of first trimester antenatal screening. *Social Science and Medicine* 61(9), pp. 1983–1992.

Chapter 5

The elephant in the consultation room

In this chapter, I explore how Down's syndrome – rather than screening itself – is constituted in prenatal care. Professionals often describe the condition, in the backstage of interviews and interactions in which parents-to-be are absent (e.g. in offices), in largely positive terms. This framing correlates with a number of their concerns, particularly that screening may amount to a 'eugenic' practice because the condition is configured, using medical discourse, as 'compatible with life'. However, such values and interpretations, and a wider discussion of Down's syndrome, are avoided and made absent in screening consultations; the condition is talked *around* as opposed to being talked *about* or *through*. This relative silence is created and upheld owing to three observations: (1) the UK public is interpreted as 'knowing' what Down's syndrome is; (2) the organisation of care dictates that the condition is not important enough to justify a detailed explanation in consultations; (3) professionals perceive themselves as having insufficient, or incomplete, knowledge of Down's syndrome. Despite professionals' worries expressed in the clinic's backstage, the condition is made absent in frontstage consultations.

Due to this explicit absence, Down's syndrome is tacitly and problematically subsumed by the broader, universalising, and negative discourse of 'risk', and ancillary categories such as 'problem' or 'abnormality', in consultations. Defining Down's syndrome as a risk, in turn, carries negative connotations; if something is a risk, it is to be feared and avoided. This helps produce and uphold the status of Down's syndrome as a negative pregnancy outcome, ensuring that familiar scripts of reproductive misfortune remain intact. In addition, such descriptions mask the huge complexity and variability of the condition, thereby silencing cultural norms and individual values which frame understandings of particular conditions. Therefore, this chapter argues that, in the clinic, professionals communicate, do not communicate, or mis-communicate information, together with power arrangements, social knowledge, and popular meanings about disability (Rapp 2000). I conclude by suggesting that screening persists since the condition is subtly constructed, in consultations and the everyday practices and relations of the clinic, as a negative outcome, ensuring that particular ways of *being* in the world are threatened and stigmatised. These claims are extended in Chapter 6.

The mundane interactions and implicit, yet deeply embedded, ideals in both Freymarsh and Springtown – figuring Down's syndrome, implicitly and it seems inadvertently, as a negative pregnancy outcome – may highlight *one* reason why termination rates for Down's syndrome have remained between 89% and 95% for over twenty years in England and Wales (Morris and Springett 2014).[1] Answering the question of why the mean rate for termination is 92% would likely be best addressed by talking to people with first-hand experience of receiving a diagnosis and having a subsequent termination of pregnancy, yet this would be expected to entail several potential pitfalls. For one, how would a researcher access such people and even if they were located, would they participate? Would delving this deep into such personal worlds constitute unethical practice? Regardless of how sensitively a study is planned, one must be cautious of the possible emotional impact on the participants (as well as the researcher). That said, there are examples of previous studies exploring how and why parents-to-be choose to terminate or continue a pregnancy after a diagnosis of Down's syndrome or other 'congenital anomaly' (Helm et al. 1998; Korenromp et al. 2007; Lotto 2015; Olarte Sierra 2010; Reist 2006; Skotko 2005; Tymstra et al. 2004) and the views of parents and siblings of people with Down's syndrome about a pregnancy termination for the condition (Ahmed et al. 2013; Bryant et al. 2005).

'Compatible with life'[2]

In Freymarsh (FAD and FMD) and Springtown (SAD), professionals convey their misgivings of Down's syndrome screening on account of its (in)accuracy and its potential to 'open a can of worms'. Another apprehension of some professionals surrounds the uncertainty of the condition (with regard to prognosis) and their view that parents-to-be have only superficial knowledge about it. A few professionals connected this to a fear that screening may satisfy a 'eugenic' function. Eugenics is defined here as practices designed to improve a population's genetic quality by pursuing the reproduction of people with desired attributes and, thus, averting the reproduction of people with undesired attributes (e.g. people with disability). Such professionals seemingly align with a definition of eugenics as the practices designed to allegedly advance society, and improve a population, by controlling reproductive practices.

The ambivalent feelings of professionals relating to the social and ethical dilemmas of reproductive technologies have been reported elsewhere (e.g. Ehrich et al. 2008). For instance, Markens (2013a; 2013b) found that genetic counsellors – whilst conveying enthusiasm for prenatal testing – show 'reflexive ambivalence', that is, they remain sceptical and concerned about the utility and consequences of parents-to-be acquiring prenatal knowledge.

Such nuanced insights seem to contradict prevalent criticisms of, and assumptions about, professionals involved in prenatal care: that they deliver a negative conception of disability by focusing largely on its physical aspects and little on the social aspects or personal experiences of disability (Farrelly et al. 2012; Lippman and Wilfond 1992). A group of respected genetic counselling veterans (Madeo et al. 2011) suggest that people in their profession do little to counteract perspectives that the lives of disabled people are judged by the very offer of screening/testing, suggesting that a more balanced view of living with disabling conditions needs to be conveyed to parents-to-be.

In addition, the troubled relationship between science, medicine, and eugenics in the context of reproductive technology has been previously recognised (Cunningham-Burley and Kerr 1999; Kerr et al. 1998; Kevles 1995), with some sceptical of the disassociation between scientific innovation and an old eugenics (Jones 1994; Shakespeare 1995). Cunningham-Burley and Kerr (1999) identify how professionals involved in genetics direct attention to the valuable social implications of intervention, rather than to the science itself, and so protect their cognitive authority whilst distancing the new genetics from charges of repeating an old eugenics. Whilst the new genetics produces and communicates neutral information offering greater choice, eugenics is framed as a feature of totalitarian regimes and a politically-distorted pseudo-science that abuses knowledge (Kerr 2003; Kerr et al. 1997).

However, in FAD and SAD, a number of professionals claim that Down's syndrome screening, a practice they are primarily responsible for, may be criticised for serving a eugenic purpose. During a conversation after an NT scan, Esther (SAD sonographer) accounts for why she believes this to be the case:

> Mr and Mrs Jansen (parents-to-be) leave. Esther comments that Mrs Jansen appeared primarily concerned with obtaining ultrasound pictures. I ask if she thinks Mrs Jansen was 'formally informed about screening':

> ESTHER: The only difference between eugenics and screening is informed consent. I have a real problem with screening for Down's [syndrome] because there's much worse out there. I fear it's eugenic. More severe conditions like Patau [syndrome] or Edward's [syndrome] are rare but not compatible with life whereas Down's is compatible with life. Everyone wants the perfect pregnancy these days. In my grandmother's generation, they didn't expect healthy babies every time. Miscarriages, stillbirths, it was expected babies wouldn't always make it. But these days, we have all the technology to know about babies and their potential problems. We've experienced a cultural shift towards perfection. [...] What makes this a non-eugenic service is the idea of getting informed consent. But informed consent is not consent at all. It's not informed if parents do it as part of the routine

of pregnancy. Parents are in a culture where they're expected to have all these tests and stuff. Scans like these and this care has been routinised so it's just consent, it's not informed consent. A number of patients still have no idea why they're in the hospital for a screen for Down's because it's so routinised and seen as what people are supposed to be doing.

Esther conveys her worry that screening is routinised since parents-to-be seemingly consent to it without great thought as 'part of the routine of pregnancy', thereby undercutting the notion of informed consent and contributing towards promoting a 'eugenic' agenda; 'the only difference between eugenics and screening is informed consent'. Current measures, for Esther, provide and promote an illusion of (informed) consent. Since parents-to-be are 'expected to have all of these tests and stuff', the notion of informed consent is farcical since they become docile and, in turn, toe the line of expectations. What makes such practices acceptable is 'the high degree of individual choice that appears to be exercised', yet 'how fragile that choice might be' is often unappreciated (Bosk 1992: 141).

Esther also identifies Patau syndrome and Edward's syndrome as 'severe' and 'rare' conditions which are 'not compatible with life'; Down's syndrome, in contrast, is 'compatible with life', leading Esther to stress that *there's much worse out there*. Here, Esther produces classifications and divisions between 'compatible' and 'non-compatible' conditions, the former becoming a catch-all term for a foetus who is 'viable' (who can live) and has a good 'quality of life'. In FAD and SAD, professionals construct Down's syndrome as 'compatible with life', commonly with reference to the separate conditions of both Edward's syndrome and Patau syndrome which are interpreted as 'incompatible with life'.[3] During a higher-risk screening consultation, for instance, Nancy (FAD midwife) defines Edward's syndrome and Patau syndrome (and Turner syndrome) as 'the nasty ones' which are 'pretty much incompatible with life'. In an interview, Amy (FAD midwife) claims that, whilst she would not terminate a pregnancy following a Down's syndrome diagnosis, she 'probably wouldn't continue with Patau [syndrome] or Edward's [syndrome]'. During an interview, Francine (FMD head midwife) suggests that diagnoses of Patau syndrome and Edward's syndrome are 'easier' for parents-to-be when they must make a decision regarding a termination following a diagnosis:

I think a misinterpretation some women have is even if they're told they've got a baby with Down's [syndrome], we'll be able to tell them what degree of Down's they have, the severity, which obviously we can't. That's very difficult because a couple may be able to cope with a mildly affected Down's baby.[4] But if they've then got behavioural problems, and cardiac issues, you can't give them that answer of to what degree the baby will be affected. Edward's [syndrome] and Patau [syndrome are] easier. The people I've counselled with abnormal results or with a higher-risk result, if they know or if they've been told that they've got a baby that's incompatible with life, it's like having your 1 in 3 chance [result of having a baby with Down's syndrome] compared to your 1 in 100. They may not decide to terminate the pregnancy but they know in the back of their minds what's likely to happen to the baby whereas with Down's, they haven't got that. It's still in that grey area.

For Francine, the uncertain prognosis of Down's syndrome – a condition that is clinically categorised as compatible with life, yet one that varies considerably between each case in relation to a person's mental and physical condition – causes problems for decision-making processes. She believes that a diagnosis of Edward's syndrome or Patau syndrome is 'easier' than a diagnosis of Down's syndrome since the latter is 'in that grey area'. This comparison to other conditions emerges in many professionals' private accounts of, and private misgivings about, screening. In her interview, Lois (FAD midwife) explains:

It is surprising we test for Down's syndrome when there are lots of things worse than it. For example, cystic fibrosis,[5] and it's something like one in twenty people are carriers. I know the risk is lower of your child having cystic fibrosis but that would be a massive thing. It shortens your life expectancy a lot more than Down's syndrome does. So I do find it surprising in a way that there's so much onus on the Down's test. But once a screening test has been introduced, it's unlikely they'd take it away.

Lois categorises cystic fibrosis as a 'massive thing' which is 'worse than' Down's syndrome, before concluding that the introduction of Down's syndrome screening prevents its withdrawal from medical practice. Amy (FAD midwife) similarly questions why Down's syndrome screening 'is highlighted because there are loads of other conditions out there that can be picked up', predicting that parents-to-be consent to it because 'they probably just feel that since the test is there and we're offering it, they should take it'. Likewise, Francine (FMD head midwife) suggests that the routinisation of screening, at the expense of 'forgetting that a child could be born with cerebral palsy or autism', shapes it as an 'anticipation engrained in them' which 'cannot be taken away because we've started it'. The most common complaint in this respect, however, is that screening for heart defects, cited in both Freymarsh and Springtown as the leading cause of death for unborn and newborn babies, is overlooked in favour of Down's syndrome screening. Dr Karman (FMD consultant) feels limited resources would be better allocated elsewhere – i.e. not to screening for Down's syndrome – given that it is 'compatible with life'. Bethan (SAD administrative staff) claims that when parents-to-be contact Springtown, she informs them that cardiac issues are more prevalent than Down's syndrome with a view to 'selling the cardiac scans'. This offer is frequently rebuffed, though, since 'it is all Down's, Down's, Down's!' During an interview, Lisa (SAD sonographer) claims:

> The NHS and a lot of people have a bee in their bonnet about Down's syndrome when the baby is far more likely to have a heart defect. But people have this big thing, like, it's terrible that the baby has Down's syndrome, whereas they're much more likely to have a baby with a heart defect. For the number of Down's syndrome babies you're detecting, they should put more money into screening for heart defects.

Lisa says that extensive screening for heart defects, seen by several professionals as a more pressing concern in prenatal care, is disregarded in favour of detecting Down's syndrome (seen as a 'terrible' outcome). Such recommendations arguably extend the medical gaze by realigning a focus on other surveillance techniques (Armstrong 1995), yet they are used here as a resource for critically reflecting on screening and the provision of services. Indeed, professionals' categorisation of Down's syndrome, with reference to other conditions and their enrolment (or not) in prenatal care, highlights one of their own ambivalences around screening. Elena (FMD head midwife), during an interview, accounts for her dislike of screening, and why:

> I think just because we can screen for Down's [syndrome], why should we? The money would be better spent elsewhere on cardiac issues and other problems. Because [people with Down's syndrome] are the gentlest, most loving people in the world. I wouldn't personally terminate a pregnancy for the condition but I wouldn't deny access to information. [...] I think Down's screening is a waste of time, effort, and money which could be well spent somewhere else for the sake of detecting how many Down's children [via prenatal testing]? And you could spend that money on giving them the most appropriate support and the family the most appropriate support you can get rather than just killing another human being because they just happen to be a bit different. I think it's just eugenics by another name. Enough is enough. I think having Down's syndrome has been demonised.

Elena, perhaps unintentionally, stumbles upon a familiar critique of prenatal testing and abortion from a disability studies perspective: if money was reallocated from prenatal screening/testing to providing more effective and accessible services to people with Down's syndrome and their families, screening/testing uptake may subsequently recede. This reflects the 'cost-benefit' analysis of screening (Saxton 2013: 93). There are enormous resources dedicated to expanding screening/testing for a few rare genetic conditions, but providing services for people with disabilities, Down's syndrome included, are likely to be significantly more costly. For Saxton, this rhetoric is problematic. First, contributions of humans cannot, and should not, be judged by how they fit into the mould of normalcy, productivity, or cost-benefit. Second, this argument distracts attention and resources from addressing the possible social and environmental causes of disability and disease. Nonetheless, for Elena, Down's syndrome screening is problematic owing to the stigmatisation ('having Down's syndrome has been demonised') and negative treatment of, and limited resources dedicated to, people living with the condition.

Elena's account is atypical in its explicit recognition of Down's syndrome screening and testing as 'killing another human being because they just happen to be a bit different', but typical in its more positive, if generalising, description of the condition itself ([people with Down's syndrome] are the gentlest, most loving people in the world'). Elena's positive image of the condition is reflected in her recognition during another conversation that Down's syndrome 'is nowhere near as bad as the other stuff', the classification of 'other stuff' denoting conditions figured as 'incompatible with life'. The following fieldnotes were taken at a multi-disciplinary team meeting[6] organised by FMD:

> Around fifteen professionals – obstetric consultants, head midwives, cardiac specialists, neurologists, and others – are in the meeting. Dr Karman begins by welcoming staff and directing their gaze to the large projector screen in FMD displaying 'cases'. [...] Dr Karman provides an update on a case where the child of a couple was postnatally diagnosed with Down's syndrome. Dr Karman informs attendees that 'they were disappointed but positive. They said "it's a shame but we'll love him anyway", so there you go.' This was met with smiles from most attendees. Some called out 'that's great' and 'good for her.'

Such meetings can provoke disagreement yet equally become a mechanism in which forms of knowing are affirmed and reproduced (Latimer 2013). In this particular meeting, professionals applaud the absent parents for their attitude to a Down's syndrome diagnosis. This echoes midwives' and sonographers' accounts when they construct a positive image of the condition, namely around its compatibility with life (whilst also acknowledging the prospective challenges of having the condition, both for an individual and their family). Even the professionals who did not openly cite this as fuelling eugenic outcomes – although, as shown, a number have – do, at the very least, express some element of trepidation about the practice relating to this knowledge. Here, their accounts seem to align with research and autobiographical accounts of parents who have a child with Down's syndrome that recognise their situation as not one which should always be viewed as unwanted and tragic (more on this later). Here, Down's syndrome is viewed as 'one way, among others, of being human' (Clarke 1994: 19).

Absence in prenatal encounters

If professionals, then, describe Down's syndrome in positive terms in the backstage of the clinic, how is it constituted in everyday affairs, that is, in screening consultations? How does it emerge in an environment that allegedly tenders little chance for people to discuss and explore their beliefs surrounding disability (Bryant et al. 2006)? Interestingly, in screening consultations in FAD and SAD, the condition is seldom addressed in explicit detail. At most, Down's syndrome is cited without any further clarification. People or things are made absent or present in everyday practices, revealing what is un/known and what is either marginalised or privileged (Rappert and Bauchspies 2014; Thomas 2016). By examining 'what is not said and who is not present' (Pascale 2011: 145) in the prenatal clinic, we can reveal what is made invisible, silenced, or made to be so taken-for-granted that it falls outside of biomedical discourse. I illustrate this point using the following fieldnotes taken during an NT scan by Esther (SAD sonographer) for Mr and Mrs Jones (parents-to-be):

ESTHER: So here's your baby. You can see the heart beating away there. Little one's hiccupping as well [Mr and Mrs Jones laugh].

MRS JONES: Maybe it's that sausage and chips I just had! [All laugh].

ESTHER: So we measure the nuchal translucency which is the pad of fluid at the back of baby's neck. When it's enlarged, it increases the risk of baby having a chromosomal abnormality. We do the measurement in combination with your blood-work so you will have some bloods done today. So the nuchal translucency and your age and your biochemical bloods and the length of the baby will give you a definite risk of three chromosomal abnormalities. We only screen for three, one of which is Down [syndrome], which I'm sure you know but also we look at Patau [syndrome] and Edward's [syndrome]. I don't know if you've seen about these on the internet but they're three of the most common, two of the most lethal. So during this screening, you'll be placed in either the lower-risk or higher-risk bracket and if you're higher-risk, you're advised to have an amniocentesis. Oh God, you've got a wriggly one in here!

MRS JONES: It looks like it's doing the splits [laughing].

ESTHER: Yes, baby's doing a dance! We like the nuchal translucency to measure less than 3mm and your measurements are all under 3mm, which is all great really.

Esther begins the scan by identifying the position and heartbeat of the foetus. Her reading of movement as 'hiccupping' means that the foetus can be viewed as an entity separate to the mother (and also by its label as a 'wriggly one'). Mrs Jones jokingly relates this to 'the sausage and chips I just had', demonstrating how Mrs Jones reclaims her and her baby as an integrated entity. Humour is littered throughout the encounter; Mr and Mrs Jones are amused by the hic-cupping which is attributed to Mrs Jones' pre-scan conduct (eating), Mrs Jones frames the movement as replicating the splits, and Esther describes the foetus as doing a dance routine. This collaborative coding reflects the intricate shifts between threat and thrill, that is, the (clinical) information communicated about screening and the (non-clinical) performance of sonographers, parents-to-be, and foetuses (Chapter 4). Threats involve divulging details of nuchal translucencies, genetic conditions, and diagnostic tests, whilst thrills involve giving parents-to-be an entertaining experience; this is indicative of, in essence, the 'humour and horror' of ultrasound (Ivry 2009: 195).

But what happens to Down's syndrome here? Throughout the consultation, whilst the condition is cited, no further details on Down's syndrome are tendered by Esther nor solicited by Mr and Mrs Jones. Assumptions appear to govern proceedings; Down's syndrome is shaped as something that the parents-to-be should 'know'. Interestingly, Esther defines the three syndromes screened for – Down's syndrome, Edward's syndrome, and Patau syndrome – as 'chromosomal abnormalities' and 'three of the most common, two of the most lethal'. Esther refrains from clarifying which syndromes are lethal, but rather relies on Mr and Mrs Jones calling on tacit assumptions regarding which conditions are lethal and which condition is not. Similar to Garfinkel's (1967) *et cetera* principle whereby people expect others to understand situations based on their own tacit knowledge, Down's syndrome is framed as a taken-for-granted category requiring no further elucidation regarding symptoms, prognosis, and 'social realities' (Rapp 1988: 150) of the child who might have the condition. The following extract is from a screening consultation between Tara (FAD midwife) and Mrs Leslie (mother-to-be):

TARA: So you know that it's a simple blood test, yes?

MRS LESLIE: Yes.

TARA: Great. We take your bloods and this will be sent off to the labs. You'll receive a letter in about seven to ten working days telling you your result. And this test goes according to your age so the older you are, the higher your risk is for having a baby with Down's syndrome.

MRS LESLIE: OK.

TARA: You will get a lower or higher-risk result. If you're lower-risk, we won't do anything else but that's not to say that there's no chance that your baby has Down's syndrome.

MRS LESLIE: Yes [nods].

TARA: If you have a higher-risk result, we'll call you up and invite you in to offer an amniocentesis. Have you had an amniocentesis before?

MRS LESLIE: No but I've heard of it.

TARA: OK. Well it's a large needle which goes into your tummy and this takes some fluid from around your baby which is sent off to be looked at. This is the test done to provide a proper diagnosis.

MRS LESLIE: Yes.

TARA: This test just tells you whether you have a higher-risk or lower-risk.

MRS LESLIE: Yes.

TARA: OK then. So you don't smoke and this isn't an IVF, no?

MRS LESLIE: No.

Tara takes more details from Mrs Leslie. After this, both Tara and Mrs Leslie leave the room so Mrs Leslie can have blood withdrawn for the quadruple screen.

The consultation begins with Tara describing screening as a 'simple blood test'. This constructs screening as a trouble-free exercise, arguably threatening the principle of non-directive care designed to govern clinical practice. By framing screening as 'simple', Tara could, albeit unwittingly, induce Mrs Leslie to undertake screening. Additionally, although Mrs Leslie's age is not explicitly cited, Tara's statement that 'the older you are, the higher your risk is for having a baby with Down's syndrome' may influence her decision. Nonetheless, my intention here is to recognise how Down's syndrome is overlooked during a consultation and lost in the trappings of clinical jargon around risk results and diagnostic testing. Here, professionals concentrate on screening processes more than the condition itself (McCourt 2006; Williams et al. 2002b).

But what about consultations whereby a Down's syndrome diagnosis is suspected after a higher-risk result is established? In such consultations, the condition is rarely afforded much attention once again. Consider the following extract taken from a consultation between Susan (FAD midwife), Mrs Garry (mother-to-be), and Mrs Garry's mother:

Susan tells Mrs Garry that she has received a 1:87 result. She explains the process which led to this 1:87 result and tells Mrs Garry that she is 'in the higher-risk group', meaning that she will be offered an amniocentesis. She explains the amniocentesis procedure whilst highlighting the 1% risk of miscarriage and other possible side effects, including abdominal cramps and heavy bleeding. Susan then explains:

SUSAN: The result will only tell you for sure about three main chromosomal abnormalities: Trisomy 21 which is Down's syndrome, Trisomy 18 which is Edward's syndrome, and Trisomy 13 which is Patau syndrome. Edward's and Patau are serious chromosomal disorders and Down's syndrome you already know about. It varies from mild through to quite severe. So this will come to you in the first three days of analysis but then the rest of your chromosomes are analysed over two weeks. This could bring out some unexpected results, even things we don't know about yet. So you could know all of these things. How do you feel about having the test?

MRS GARRY: I'd be more worried if it was a 1 in 30 result. But it's 1 in 87 isn't it?

SUSAN: Yes. The number does make a difference. [Mrs Garry looks anxious] It's totally up to you. You don't have to decide today. You have to consider your feelings and then decide.

Mrs Garry's mother asks how long they can wait before Mrs Garry can decide whether to have an amniocentesis. Susan explains that there is currently an available timeslot for amniocentesis in two days' time. Mrs Garry says she will not accept this timeslot yet and will go home to discuss options with her partner. Susan accepts this, hands Mrs Garry a leaflet on having a higher-risk result, and says Mrs Garry can telephone her at any time if she has any questions. Mrs Garry asks questions such as 'who usually has amniocentesis' (Susan specifies 'it's totally up to you') and claims the result was 'not as high as I was expecting anyway'. She asks if the anomaly scan can detect Down's syndrome (Susan answers it might if there is a heart defect) and if there is a timescale for deciding whether to have amniocentesis:

SUSAN: Not really. But we do say it's better to have it sooner as it'll get harder to make that decision as the pregnancy goes on and you start to feel the baby kick and stuff.

MRS GARRY: So the sooner the better really?

SUSAN: Yes. But take your time in making the decision. We can do whatever you need us to do.

Susan asks if Mrs Garry has any more questions. She does not. Mrs Garry and her mother thank Susan before leaving the room.

After describing to Mrs Garry how she is 'in the higher-risk group', Susan asks her how she feels about the test and reiterates that this decision is to be made by her and her partner. Susan explains that a timeslot for amniocentesis has been booked, arguably dismissing the principle of non-directive care. Intimating that the gravity of the situation requires immediate attention could have an effect of implicitly coercing Mrs Garry to have the procedure. Arguably, such claims are a form of pastoral power which governs bodies and organises actions (Foucault 1979). Power relations are enacted subtly here, encouraging Mrs Garry to – or at best advising her to – conduct herself in a particular way. This is reinforced by Susan suggesting that whilst Mrs Garry has full jurisdiction in deciding if/when she would like an amniocentesis, it would be 'better to have it sooner as it'll get harder to make that decision', a decision presumably regarding a termination of pregnancy, 'as the pregnancy goes on and you start to feel the baby kick and stuff'.

An important observation here involves Susan's explanation that an amniocentesis can initially provide a diagnosis of Down's syndrome, Edward's syndrome, or Patau syndrome. She also states that the test can 'bring out some unexpected results, even things we don't know yet' – the 'dragnet' effect of screening that can thrust mothers-to-be into decision-making processes that were not expected when first consenting (Alderson et al. 2004: 75). Susan describes Edward's syndrome and Patau syndrome as 'serious chromosomal disorders'; in contrast, Down's syndrome is figured as something that Mrs Garry 'already know[s] about' and which 'varies from mild through to quite severe'. Again, no more details about Down's syndrome are given. In consultations, attention is focused instead on the designation of a risk factor, diagnostic testing, and the timescale of decision-making processes. Here, Down's syndrome becomes an example of absence in prenatal medicine (Latimer and Thomas 2015). It is comparable to Latour's (1999: 304) 'black box', a metaphor referring to how 'scientific and technical work is made invisible by its own success'. Latour argues that the complexity of a given system's internal workings is redundant providing that it continues to serve its primary purpose and allows people to proceed in their daily activities. The inner workings of a black box are not open for debate as it has been accepted by the scientific community and society alike. Its output, therefore, retains the status of truth. Whilst Latour's description shows how scientific facts are established, I suggest that, within screening, the medical category of Down's syndrome becomes a black box, a known entity that often remains closed; professionals do not provide, nor do parents solicit or question, details about it. To take another metaphor, it becomes an elephant in the (consultation) room. In what follows, I unpack how the black box of Down's syndrome is solidified and darkened, who is involved in this, what affects this has, and why this is significant when reflecting on the politics of prenatal care.

Accounting for absence

So why is Down's syndrome absent within consultations? I provide three possible reasons for this: (1) the familiarity of Down's syndrome; (2) the organisation of care; (3) professionals' knowledge of the condition. I expand on each of these points below.

'A public secret': the familiarity of Down's syndrome

As alluded to in one of the extracts above (Esther and Mr and Mrs Jones), Down's syndrome constitutes a taken-for-granted category that is recognisable to parents-to-be. Professionals suggest that the general public, at large, know about Down's syndrome – but that this knowledge is limited to anatomical features, or the 'face' (Latimer 2013: 12), of the condition. During an interview, Amy (FAD midwife) explains:

> I don't think expectant parents understand Down's syndrome much
> unless they have a family member or a friend who has a Down's syndrome

person in the family. But I think they know what a Down's syndrome person looks like. They don't always know a Down's syndrome person can live until they're sixty-five and seventy [years old] and can live a relatively normal life in the sense that they get up in the morning, eat and dress, and that.

Amy doubts whether the majority of parents-to-be hold detailed knowledge about the condition, such as the life expectancy of individuals with Down's syndrome and their capacity to 'live a relatively normal life'. Amy, and others, feel that parents-to-be are not fully aware of key features of Down's syndrome, a trend reported elsewhere (Bryant et al. 2006; Ternby et al. 2015b; Williams et al. 2002a; 2002b; 2002c), and that this undermines 'informed' choice. However, they are described as knowing 'what someone with Down's syndrome looks like' owing to the distinctive facial features caused by the presence of an extra chromosome. Susan and Maggie (FAD midwives), and others, credit an awareness of this 'face' to the familiar presence of people with the condition in the UK. In an interview, Camilla (FAD midwife) explains the difficulties of communicating information to parents-to-be whose first language is not English:

> You often get women from other countries that don't speak English as a first language and maybe don't really understand what a baby with Down's syndrome is because of language barriers and cultural differences. Whether they really understand what we're asking of them or what we're trying to explain in consultations, I'm not convinced. Some people do say 'I don't know what a Down's syndrome baby is.' And you think, gosh, really [laughs]?

For Camilla, 'language barriers and cultural differences' may lessen the knowledge of parents-to-be with respect to Down's syndrome; local metaphors of pregnancy, birth, and parenthood do not easily translate 'into the realm of medical discourse' (Rapp 2000: 81). During consultations in FAD and SAD, regardless of the language proficiency of parents-to-be, Down's syndrome was rarely explicated in any detail. Considering that 'it helps to know about Down's syndrome as this would affect whether [parents-to-be] have the screening or not', as Lois (FAD midwife) identifies, and professionals worry that parents-to-be only have a superficial grasp of the condition (namely, common facial features), why are no further details offered? Susan (FAD midwife), among others, admits to 'not speaking about Down's syndrome' but why is this so?

One reason for this is that the familiarity of the Down's syndrome 'face' hinders a broader discussion of the condition. A second reason, possibly, is that parents-to-be and professionals do not want to consider it as a possible pregnancy outcome. Lisa (SAD sonographer) says during an interview that this is because Down's syndrome is principally understood in negative terms:

I think [parents-to-be] probably see [Down's syndrome] as very negative by and large. I don't think they know how much support they would get or if they're told what life would be like if they're given the diagnosis of a Down's syndrome baby. How much they're told will influence them whether they'd keep the pregnancy or not.

Whilst Lisa's contentions relate to terminating or continuing a pregnancy following a diagnosis, her claims are appropriate for considering how Down's syndrome is constituted in the early stages of prenatal care. Elena (FMD head midwife) conveys a similar thought, saying that 'people's understandings' reflect stereotypes such as 'the older person walking behind their elderly parents with the ankle socks'. The following fieldnotes were taken in the Springtown office where parents-to-be book ultrasound scans:

Dominique, Juliana, and Hannah (administrative staff) discuss the nuchal translucency scan.

GARETH: Do you think expectant parents having the nuchal translucency scan know much about Down's syndrome?
DOMINIQUE: Not really. I think they know about the facial features.
HANNAH: I don't think they want to know.
DOMINIQUE: It's not fully entered their heads.
JULIANA: And they know about them being retarded.[7]
DOMINIQUE: I don't think they know because it's such a broad spectrum of how they are affected too.
HANNAH: Unless they know of someone in the family.
JULIANA: We get more questions about Patau syndrome and Edward's syndrome. With these syndromes, they ask things like 'What are they?' Because they aren't as well-known so we tell them about that and that's it really. We bracket it in with Down's syndrome.

Dominique casts doubt on whether parents-to-be know about Down's syndrome, excusing 'facial features', because the condition had 'not fully entered their heads' and there is 'such a broad spectrum of how they are affected'. Juliana suspects that parents-to-be will likely know about people with Down's syndrome having learning difficulties and so ask 'more questions about Patau syndrome and Edward's syndrome', two conditions 'bracket[ed] in with Down's syndrome', as these are not 'as well known'. Importantly, Hannah explains that parents-to-be do not have much knowledge of the condition since 'I don't think they want to know'. Returning to screening consultations, silence seems to act as some sort of barrier, with interaction being carefully orchestrated to mask certain conversations. It is feasible to contend that the imagined damage caused by the potential presence of a baby with Down's syndrome, as a future deviant body, initiates reluctance from both parties to openly thrash out the details of the condition. This silence may also be interpreted as professionals attempting to reduce anxiety among parents-to-be. The topic of Down's syndrome may be averted due to a sense of 'jinx' – by naming the threat, it is somehow more likely to happen. This mirrors the claims of others who suggest that professionals withhold some information from parents-to-be about possible pregnancy outcomes to avoid causing any needless angst (Burton-Jeangros et al. 2013; Ivry 2006).

In addition, professionals may not discuss Down's syndrome in any great detail since they have little to offer other than a description of the variability and unpredictability of expression (professional knowledge is discussed later in this chapter). As such, in Freymarsh and Springtown, the condition is subjected to 'civil inattention' (Goffman 1971: 126) where professionals and parents-to-be dis-attend to the condition. As an elephant in the room, it amounts to what Taussig (1999: 7) describes as a 'public secret', namely the ideas of shared knowledge in a society that is seldom described or explicitly acknowledged. Symbolically invisible and at its core banal, public secrets become a powerful social glue and knowledge of 'knowing what not to know' (1999: 6). Rarely were such secrets defaced in the clinic's frontstage (but discussions did take place in the clinic's backstage, as conveyed earlier in this chapter). At the crossroads between the unmentioned and unmentionable, Down's syndrome is exposed to a strange yet pervasive 'degradation ceremony' (Garfinkel 1956: 420) and is downgraded through its silence. It is in its familiarity that Down's syndrome, curiously, becomes invisible.

The organisation of care

A second reason why Down's syndrome remains absent from consultations is that the organisation of care hinders interactions between parents-to-be and professionals. This is most applicable in FAD where a checklist is used to govern clinical practice when doing Down's syndrome screening (this check-list is not used at SAD). It includes eleven 'key points to discuss', in Camilla's (FAD midwife) words, in a consultation:

> After a consultation, Camilla fills in a checklist. The first side of the form asks for details such as scan date, ethnic origin, and weight. The second side contains a list of 11 points marked 'Information Given' which must be clarified during consultations:
>
> 1   Gestation at the time of test
> 2   Have you had any other screening test for Down's syndrome?
> 3   A low chance result ≥ 1:151
> 4   Low chance does not mean no chance
> 5   Low chance result will be sent by letter within 10 working days
> 6   The low chance letter will not state the risk ratio

7   A high chance result ≤ 1:150
8   High chance screening result will be provided within five working days
9   An appointment will be offered within 24 hours of contact to discuss a high chance result
10   Have you considered the amniocentesis test that will be offered following a high chance result?
11   If you accept an amniocentesis diagnostic test an appointment will be offered as soon as possible following a recall.

Camilla suggests that 'in order to cover our backs', professionals follow such rationalised stipulations with the intention of accomplishing appropriate care and avoiding possible litigation. The checklist was introduced about 6–7 months into fieldwork at Freymarsh. I was told that the reason for this was that a mother, who was screened for Down's syndrome at FAD, threatened legal action after receiving a 'lower-risk result' but giving birth to a child with the condition. The checklist was subsequently introduced as a measure in order to try to prevent this from happening again. Martha (FAD midwife) discusses its value during an interview:

It makes sure we're all practising to the same standard so that one midwife doesn't go in and just skip through it. It standardises practice. With other things you can't be all the same but with screening for Down's syndrome, what we say should be standardised before the screening is done.

Lindsay (FAD midwife) similarly claims that the new checklist is 'making a difference' and that parents-to-be 'might not assume it's just a blood test and that people just have it'. Likewise, Lois (FAD midwife) explains that many aspects of prenatal care are reduced to 'tick-boxing, initialling, and that's it', citing this as a positive development in the 'streamlining' of tasks so there is not 'too much paperwork'. Rita (FAD midwife) explains that she also likes the checklist since 'you've got it all there ready to remind you' and claims that the consultation is 'just tick'; her care, thus, is accomplished by ticking the specified boxes. The checklist is an 'immutable mobile' (Latour 1987: 237), a textual form which represents knowledge and remains constant as it flows through various networks. For Latour, immutable mobiles are crucial to routinising scientific knowledge and techniques. The immutable mobile of the screening checklist is translated into practical situations (consultations) and whilst subject to reinterpretation, is dutifully followed by FAD midwives with the intention of providing informed choice. The checklist also represents a response to potential lawsuits; by communicating all of the 'correct' information at hand, midwives 'back-up' by engaging in 'defensive practice' (Gail, FAD midwife).

The checklist is framed positively as it specifies the important data requiring explication. This also reflects the routinisation and rationalisation of care/screening practices. Press and Browner (1997) argue that the relatively banal way in which prenatal screening is presented causes it to become a routine practice among other procedures. Returning to the checklist, a conversation about Down's syndrome does not constitute a 'key point to discuss'. With care increasingly structured on rational grounds in the pursuit of efficiency, and with professionals operating within strict time constraints, standardised stipulations introduced by organisational cultures determine what information is deemed necessary for sharing with parents-to-be (Bosk 1992). Conformity to rationalised modes of care shaped by wider organisational cultures – meaning that care is, essentially, read off the page – arguably limits an extensive dialogue between each party about Down's syndrome. Although the checklist is exclusive to FAD, the absence of Down's syndrome during consultations in SAD can also be attributed to an extensive deliberation of the condition being framed as non-essential or, rather, as not quite making the cut within time-limited encounters. Professionals follow a 'script' (though not a physical script – as with the checklist) that is similarly standardised, with professionals frequently conveying the same information throughout each separate consultation (in Chapter 3, this is identified as one reason for screening being downgraded, namely, that consultations can be monotonous).

It is worth returning to arguments in Chapter 4 here, where I described how professionals quash their own reservations and unease with screening by privileging the rhetoric of informed choice and non-directive care. The checklist (FAD) and verbal script (SAD) for conducting screening consultations equally show that professionals responsible for delivering this programme, and guided by organisational principles, must undertake serious behind-the-scenes (moral) labour. They silence their beliefs, ambiguities, and, at times, outright criticisms to accommodate personal values with their professional position and, thus, be able to carry out their daily work. Importantly, this silencing is so strong that slippage was rarely, if ever, observed during screening consultations between professionals and parents-to-be. Since care is confined within the rigid parameters of the checklist and the script, values and bias are silenced and, in turn, so too is Down's syndrome.

Knowledge of Down's syndrome

A third reason for the absence of Down's syndrome in consultations relates to professionals' knowledge of the condition. Whilst several midwives and sonographers feel that they have a good knowledge of Down's syndrome, others admit to lacking extensive knowledge of it. Asked about the knowledge of parents-to-be regarding Down's syndrome, Sophie (SAD sonographer) says:

> I think a lot of them probably don't really know about [Down's syndrome]. I suppose it's just what you read about or people or families you know. [...] I must admit we haven't particularly been taught a lot about

it. I know a lot about testing for it but I don't know a huge amount about the actual condition. I think it goes back to if you know somebody with it and we're taught things like the statistics, like 25% of them can have cardiac problems. But you're not particularly taught about that when you do training and stuff.

After suspecting that parents-to-be do not know much about the condition, Sophie associates her limited knowledge with a lack of training and suggests that her familiarity with it relates exclusively to screening practices and statistics ('25% of them have cardiac problems'). According to several sources, however, the number of people with Down's syndrome who have cardiac issues is closer to 50% (NHS FASP 2012). The argument that professionals involved in screening have varying and often low levels of knowledge of Down's syndrome, and that medical training includes little direct contact with people with developmental disabilities, is outlined elsewhere (Cleary-Goldman et al. 2006; Driscoll et al. 2009; Skirton and Barr 2010; Skotko 2005; Ternby et al. 2015a). Francine (FMD head midwife) reflects on this lack of knowledge during an interview whilst discussing her daily work in FMD:

> I feel that in FMD, we are treated well by parents-to-be because they are sent to us having seen midwives or doctors [outside of FMD]. And quite a lot of the time, the midwives and doctors will give them the very basic information and refer them here because most midwives and doctors don't like abnormalities. It's not in their realm of interest or knowledge so if an abnormality comes, I mean that is the best way because it's better not to explain if you don't know what you're talking about rather than giving information we're potentially going to contradict.

Francine suggests that midwives and doctors outside of FMD 'will give [parents-to-be] the very basic information' and 'do not like abnormalities'. Yet it is primarily FAD midwives (and SAD sonographers) who communicate information on Down's syndrome in the early stages of prenatal care. During a conversation in the office, Rita (FAD midwife) highlights the difficulties of explaining a condition without extensive knowledge of it:

> Even if you get a result that means expectant parents will be referred elsewhere, you're the initial person to see them. Sometimes I find that a bit difficult because they start asking you questions and I cannot always answer them because I'm not specialised in that area. So I feel a bit bad then saying 'I'm not really the best person to speak to but I will get someone to speak to you'.

Rita describes how it is 'a bit difficult' when parents-to-be 'start asking questions' which 'I cannot always answer because I'm not specialised in the area'. Such observations implicitly reflect how Down's syndrome screening is downgraded in the clinic. The organisational structure dictates that screening is cast as a mundane task relegated by professionals highly placed in a clinical hierarchy (Chapter 3). Screening consultations are, instead, done by professionals who may not always, by their own admission, possess extensive knowledge of the condition; Down's syndrome, thus, becomes absent.

Notably, the condition may be afforded further details and reflection once a diagnosis is suspected and a higher-risk result must be explained to parents-to-be in another consultation (to repeat, this follows the initial screening consultation and involves asking parents-to-be if they want diagnostic testing). However, similar to initial screening consultations, most encounters are carried out by midwives in FAD (SAD sonographers bestow this responsibility to a nurse or administrative staff). During a consultation in which Mr and Mrs Knight (parents-to-be) are told that they have a higher risk of Down's syndrome, for instance, Eve and Amy (FAD midwives) describe what will happen after diagnostic testing:

> EVE: If the baby is diagnosed with Down's syndrome, you can wait until your full karyotype is in to see whether it's mild or severe.
>
> MR KNIGHT: What is severe then?
>
> EVE: I couldn't tell you that. Not now anyway.
>
> MRS KNIGHT: I think what my husband is asking is what would mild be?
>
> EVE: Well, a number of people with Down's syndrome can go on to live until sixty years old, and [Eve seems unsure and pauses].
>
> AMY: Yes, they can sometimes have learning difficulties. But if mild, they can appear quite normal.
>
> EVE: Yes. They can have a similar IQ level to other children. They can live good lives, some can live independently. [Eve pauses again] It depends really.
>
> MR KNIGHT: I do have another different question: Where does Down's syndrome start?
>
> MRS KNIGHT: Where it's from?
>
> EVE: It's an extra chromosome. That chromosome will be placed some-where in the genes. We're not sure why it happens.
>
> MR KNIGHT: I read it was when the cells were divided in the chromosomes.
>
> AMY: It's a chromosomal thing, yes. It's not genetic.
>
> MRS KNIGHT: [Turning to Mr Knight] There's nothing we can do about it, it's not one of us.
>
> EVE: Yes it's not a genetic thing.
>
> AMY: Yes.
>
> EVE: It's a chromosomal thing.

It is rare that two midwives are present during a consultation, either for Down's syndrome screening or delivering higher-risk results. On this occasion, Amy was with Eve as a training exercise (Chapter 3: 'see one, do one'). During such encounters, professionals discuss several issues with parents-to-be, including the meaning of risk factors, the benefits/risks of diag-nostic testing, and possible outcomes if a diagnosis is established (continuing or terminating a pregnancy). This information is repeated in leaflets distributed to parents-to-be at the end of the procedure. If they decide to pursue diagnostic testing, more leaflets are provided during this consultation about amniocent-esis/CVS before undertaking the procedure. A higher-risk result often causes parents-to-be to ask further questions about diagnostic testing and risk factors in a consultation. Throughout this encounter, Mr and Mrs Knight ask ques-tions regarding Down's syndrome, one of which surrounds its causes. Yet, in most consultations of this nature, a discussion of the condition rarely extends beyond midwives or other professionals offering parents-to-be a leaflet.

In Springtown, the written information provided to parents following a higher-risk result does not refer to Down's syndrome; it is limited to infor-mation on amniocentesis and its risks, blood group types, what parents should do before and after the test, and when a result will be received. In contrast, the Freymarsh leaflet does offer further details on Down's syndrome, specifi-cally how it is a 'lifelong condition which will result in some degree of learning disability'. It also highlights how the cause of Down's syndrome is unclear ('it is not known what makes this happen'), the common symptoms and prognosis of the condition ('slanted eyes', 'looser muscles and joints than other babies', 'children usually develop and learn more slowly than other children', 'they may have some medical problems that need special attention and treatments'), and existing support services for parents. This description is balanced with more positive discourse relating to early prognosis ('most children will learn to walk and talk [...] go to mainstream schools and learn to read and write') and later life ('most children and adults can lead healthy lives', 'adults can live partly-independent lives, choosing their friends and partners and working or contributing to society in other ways'). This seems to con-tradict earlier studies arguing that leaflets for Down's syndrome screening contain false, misleading, and inconsistent information on the condition (Bryant et al. 2001; Murray et al. 2001). Even so, a familiar concern of pro-fessionals in Freymarsh and Springtown is that parents-to-be rarely read the literature. If true, the non-discussion of Down's syndrome in consultations becomes even more significant.

The case cited above (with Eve, Amy, and Mr and Mrs Knight) is atypical, a 'breach' (Garfinkel 1967) or 'infraction' (Goffman 1971), as the parents-to-be *do* solicit details from the midwives in a manner that unmasks the elephant in the room. Eve and Amy (particularly Eve) seem unsure about the condition and subsequently provide vague information. Towards the consultation's conclusion, Eve and Amy, providing what could be perceived as a rather positive outlook of the condition, describe Down's syndrome as chromosomal but 'not a genetic thing'. The parents-to-be interpret the condition, then, as non-hereditary[8] and as something that they can 'do [nothing] about', thus alleviating any possible guilt further down the line that Mr Knight or Mrs Knight were (genetically) responsible for a diagnosis (Arribas-Ayllon et al. 2008; Löwy 2014). Here, there is a lack of knowledge of Down's syndrome as 'not genetic' – although Mr and Mrs Knight correctly interpret this as signifying hereditariness, reflecting popular interpretations confusing 'genetic' and 'hereditary' – and of people with the condition as 'sometimes' having learning difficulties (they will always have a cognitive impairment, although its severity and meaning is open to variation and interpretation). In addition, Eve's claim that 'you can wait until your full karyotype is in to see whether [the diagnosis is] mild or severe' seems mistaken, since the severity of Down's syndrome cannot be predicted on the basis of karyotyping. On rare occasions where information on Down's syndrome is shared or solicited, professionals commonly admit to lacking great knowledge of the condition (outside of the 'face', possible heart defects, learning difficulties, viability, chromosomal origins, and uncertain prognosis). In addition, the finer details of symptoms, prognosis, and future prospects – physiological and social – are absent or, at best, vaguely present in consultations.

My intention here is certainly not to shame or chastise professionals for their varying, or low, levels of knowledge pertaining to Down's syndrome. This knowledge is not attributable to ineptitude but, rather, is a product of relegating (and subsequently downgrading) screening to professionals who may not always have a clear grasp of the condition. This identifies possible future training needs for professionals as their current knowledge may curb opportunities for meaningful and productive conversations with parents-to-be. That said, professionals do not necessarily view a lack of knowledge about Down's syndrome, despite its wide availability (e.g. using the internet), as a deficit in performing clinical duties. The importance of professionals' knowledge about Down's syndrome and other conditions for reproductive decision-making is emphasised by others (Boardman 2010; Bryant et al. 2001; García et al. 2012; Skirton and Barr 2007). However, in FAD and SAD, the absence of Down's syndrome becomes a natural and enduring condition and, as such, a negative conception of the condition – highlighted by professionals who claim that public attitudes to the condition are largely negative – remains intact.

Risks, problems, and abnormalities

So with the condition spoken *around* as opposed to spoken *about*, what existing discourses shape Down's syndrome in interactional exchanges in the clinic? How is the condition discussed when, in turn, it is not discussed? The most common vernacular that organises and configures Down's syndrome, a vernacular infiltrating prenatal screening practices (Heyman et al. 2006; Pilnick 2008) and prenatal care more widely (Possamai-Inesedy 2006), is 'risk': parents-to-be receive a risk factor, diagnostic testing carries a risk of miscarriage (as well as heavy bleeding, abdominal cramps, infection, and premature labour), and older mothers-to-be are at an increased risk of having a child with Down's syndrome. Screening, indeed, furthers a culture of risk within the clinic in which professionals and parents-to-be must embrace complex risk assessments before the latter decide whether to undertake screening (and perhaps diagnostic testing) and assess the ultimate value of this intervention (Hallowell 1999; Rapp 2000).

In a trend reflecting the development of 'biomedicalisation' (Clarke et al. 2003), reproductive medicine positions mothers-to-be in a web of surveillance wherein they monitor, measure, and seek knowledge of avoidable 'risks' during a pregnancy (Helén 2005). Lupton (1999: 60) identifies how pregnant women are subjected to advice and appraisal directed at 'containing risks', both those threatening their health and that of the foetus. Female bodies, particularly, are 'constructed and experienced through discourses, knowledges and strategies of risk' (1999: 61). Since childbearing is a public as well as private activity, pregnant women become vulnerable to advice, criticism, and surveillance in which they are subtly disciplined into rationalising their conduct. In a risk-averse culture, pregnancy involves heavily prescriptive (moral) codes of expected conduct that are administered via a scrutinising public gaze (Lupton 1999). In FAD and SAD, for instance, mothers-to-be are burdened with information on various 'risks' including car safety, airline travel (DVT[9]), consumption (caffeine, alcohol, cigarettes, diet), sex, exercise, breastfeeding, chicken pox, flu vaccines, and gardening (exposure to toxoplasmosis/manure).

During screening for Down's syndrome at FAD and SAD, risk is an accepted and privileged discourse, the commitment to which is exemplified in the following consultation between Lois (FAD midwife) and Mrs Roberts (mother-to-be):

LOIS: This is just a chat about the Down's syndrome test. Do you know much about Down's syndrome screening?

MRS ROBERTS: Not really. I know if it's abnormal, they'll offer me another test.

LOIS: Kind of. Do you know what Down's syndrome is?

MRS ROBERTS: Yes.

LOIS: OK. This is a screening test which won't affect the baby. You'll be placed in a higher-risk or lower-risk category. The test is 80% accurate so low-risk does not mean no risk of having a baby with Down's syndrome. If you're higher-risk, we'll offer you an amniocentesis. The cut off is 1 in 150 so you could be 1 in 148, 1 in 149, 1 in 150, and all that is higher-risk. So we offer the amniocentesis which takes fluid from around the baby and this says for definite whether your baby has an abnormality. But it does have a risk of miscarriage of 1% so if 1 in 100 women have the amniocentesis, one will miscarry. A higher-risk result will be given in five working days and an appointment will be offered within twenty-four hours. A lower-risk result will be given within ten working days and the letter will say how low-risk you are. But what I badly need to know is whether you want to know whether you're a lower-risk or higher-risk.

MRS ROBERTS: Yes, just so I can know.

LOIS: So you would consider having the amniocentesis?

MRS ROBERTS: I'm not sure. I'd have to speak to my partner.

LOIS: But you'd like to know whether you're lower-risk or higher-risk?

MRS ROBERTS: Yes. I can do something about it afterwards then if something is wrong.

The consultation is described by Lois as 'just a chat', possibly becoming – as outlined in Chapter 3 – 'just another blood test' (Press and Browner 1997: 984). This can be interpreted as an effort to manage the anxiety of Mrs Roberts. However, an effect of describing the consultation in this way is that it implicitly and immediately downplays the significance of the event. Importantly, after Mrs Roberts confirms that she knows what Down's syndrome is, no further details on the condition are offered. It retains its status as 'abnormal', an unchallenged label offered by Mrs Roberts and one Lois later assumes. Lois also describes the screen as physically unproblematic ('this is a screening test which won't affect the baby'), glossing over the prospective 'can of worms' (as outlined by midwives and sonographers earlier in the book) which screening practices threaten to expose. Lois recounts what she perceives as apt information for accomplishing appropriate care, such as the accuracy of screening, risk factor cut-off rates, prospective diagnostic testing, and the risk of miscarriage (as outlined in the screening checklist discussed above). Notably, although diagnostic testing risks (e.g. miscarriage) are not explicitly outlined on the checklist discussed above, this is regularly mentioned in consultations with respect to point 10: 'Have you considered the amniocentesis test that will be offered following a high chance result?'.

The consultation is not always 'a chat' (a chat implies an inclusive two-way exchange), as described at the start of the encounter, with Lois one-sidedly reciting clinically correct information with the intention of promising the ideals of reproductive choice and non-directive care (Chapter 4). In addition, the offer of an amniocentesis 'within twenty-four hours' highlights the gravity of the situation. Similar attempts to swiftly book diagnostic tests were observed in Freymarsh, sometimes occurring before professionals informed parents-to-be of their higher-risk result. Provisional bookings are scheduled both for practical purposes (to save time in a busy environment) and for 'care' purposes (so that they could inform parents-to-be that a timeslot for diagnostic testing is available should they want it). However, whilst such actions are meant to be harmless, they could arguably coerce parents-to-be into making particular decisions (amniocentesis) and timely decisions (e.g. provisional bookings). Although hurrying the mother-to-be into making a decision may be defined as 'good care', it can also be construed as another system of disciplinary power (Foucault 1973).

After Lois asks Mrs Roberts whether she wants screening, she claims she will 'just so [she] can know', in her words, 'if something is wrong'. Importantly for the claims being made here, it is clear during the consultation that Lois uses the word risk on several occasions. The implicit assumptions shaping wider readings of risk paint a negative picture. A potential risk status not only shifts health(y) identities of mothers-to-be but also demarcates Down's syndrome itself as a 'risk', in effect, a threatening possibility. Pregnancies become 'tentative' (Rothman 1986), marred by the risk of impending disability and provoking anxiety rather than reassurance for parents-to-be (Marteau 1995). Although Lois and Mrs Roberts each define the condition as 'abnormal'/an 'abnormality', the word 'risk' principally shapes their understandings here. With Down's syndrome lacking a language of its own, it becomes subsumed by the 'linguistically and culturally more secure notion of risk' (Scamell and Alaszewski 2012: 218). The widely circulated term *risk* carries negative connotations; if something is a risk, it is to be feared and avoided (Douglas 1992; Lupton and Tulloch 2002). Since risk has 'connotations of danger and negative outcomes' (Shakespeare 1999: 673), describing Down's syndrome as a risk produces a portrayal of it as a negative, and preventable, conclusion to a pregnancy. Once more, professionals' positive configurations that emerged in the backstage of the clinic are made absent in frontstage consultations, with risk being the prevailing discourse for constituting Down's syndrome.

Interestingly, the use of the term *risk* was challenged by midwives and sonographers in both Freymarsh and Springtown and by governing bodies administering stipulations for best clinical practice. Members of each party suggest that the term *chance* should be embraced over *risk* in consultations; parents-to-be, for instance, should be told that they receive a chance result, as opposed to a risk result, of having a child with Down's syndrome (notably, the checklist outlined above uses the term *chance*). During one conversation, Amy and Gail (FAD midwives) reflect on why this is the case, with Amy concluding that 'risk sounds too negative'. During another conversation, Amy describes the word risk as 'aggressive terminology', with chance being seen as 'softer' and not sounding 'as much like a danger'. By highlighting during an interview how risk 'is negative' and that 'low-risk and high-risk is not the nicest way of saying a result', Camilla (FAD midwife) says that she tells parents-to-be that the test will 'put you into one of two groups: one that we offer you the amniocentesis and one where we don't' since risk factors/statistics 'can confuse people sometimes'.

The discourse of chance is favoured by professionals not only because it is viewed as less aggressive than risk but also since, perhaps, it implicitly attributes a result to fate/luck. Whilst risk holds connotations with danger and as something to be minimised or avoided with due attention, chance is synonymous with luck and fate. This potentially absolves parents-to-be (and particularly mothers-to-be) from feelings of responsibility for not preventing such a risk. However, my observational work reveals that, whilst both terms were occasionally used synonymously, *risk* is used far more frequently than *chance* in screening consultations. This oversight did not appear to emerge as a conscious decision but, rather, as a product of the integration of a risk discourse into the everyday work of professionals.

Within screening practices, the figuring of the condition as a risk is reinforced with similar classifications. At Freymarsh and Springtown, Down's syndrome – as it is not cited explicitly – becomes synonymous with 'problems', 'bad news', 'a bad scenario', 'something wrong', and, most frequently, 'abnormality'. The following fieldnotes taken from an NT scan by Olivia (SAD sonographer) for Mr and Mrs Burton (parents-to-be) highlight this:

> OLIVIA: Now the nuchal translucency involves measuring the fluid at the back of the baby's neck. This white line and this white line is where it is. We want that gap to be less than 3mm and I can say it looks tiny from first view.
>
> MRS BURTON: So that's a good one?
>
> OLIVIA: Yes.
>
> MRS BURTON: So it's a bad scenario if the bit at the back of the neck is not there then?
>
> OLIVIA: No. The more it is, the higher the chance of abnormality. So a small measurement is good. The measurement is 1.6mm too which is brilliant.

In this consultation, Olivia repairs the impending danger of a 'bad scenario' by highlighting the 'brilliant' measurement which, in all likelihood, points toward the absence not of Down's syndrome but of the vaguer category of 'abnormality'. The nuchal translucency is categorised as a 'good one', with most foetuses being 'normal' and falling under the rubric of 'nice news'. Despite this reassurance being present in most consultations, a commitment to discursive categories of risks, problems, and bad scenarios takes on greater significance once you consider Francine's (FMD head midwife) suspicion that parents-to-be 'only really pick up keywords'. Since professional conduct incites interpretive acts among parents-to-be, the discursive categories tendered by professionals classify Down's syndrome as a negative outcome. Furthermore, it imposes a collective category on Down's syndrome which blurs the considerable variation, not only of the condition, but also between two or more people with the condition (Thomas and Rothman 2016). This corresponds to the claims of the disability movement that screening and aborting a foetus diagnosed with a condition, such as Down's syndrome, is a 'major component of the forms of discrimination that create disability' (McLaughlin 2003: 298; see also: Shakespeare 1998; 2006).

The masking of the variability of Down's syndrome in terms of expression, specifically with respect to the categorical work (Bowker and Star 2000) of professionals, is examined further in Chapter 6. At this point, I recognise that, whilst Down's syndrome is a complex and heterogeneous condition with symptoms varying significantly in each case, it is also not a benign condition; symptoms can be debilitating and, in some cases, fatal. However, the intention is to highlight that, irrespective of *what* particular effects Down's syndrome may have for someone born with the condition, the categories of risk, problem, or abnormality act as a stiff mould that may conceal certain variations (e.g. physiological and intellectual) and intricacies. This is made clear in parents-to-be being offered screening, at once, for several conditions and diseases including, but not limited to, rubella, HIV, syphilis, rhesus disease,[10] sickle-cell disease,[11] thalassemia,[12] hepatitis B/C, and Down's syndrome. During an interview, Maggie (FAD midwife) describes the impact that this may have on parents-to-be:

> I think most people just assume [Down's syndrome screening] is something they're going to have. It's like we check their blood, their iron levels, we check their blood group, and we'll check their Down's syndrome blood at the same time. It's very common now. Everyone just takes it.

Maggie describes how the naturalisation of Down's syndrome screening can be attributed to parents-to-be assuming that screening is 'something they're going to have' together with other tests. Rita (FAD midwife) similarly says that screening is accepted by parents-to-be since it is offered together with screening for the likes of rubella and hepatitis B. She feels that Down's syndrome screening, perceived as 'routine and what [parents-to-be] do', should be 'separated from the rest of them', criticising current practice for not formulating distinctions between the former and the latter. Both Maggie and Rita, together with other professionals, acknowledge this trend to highlight the problem of Down's syndrome screening being framed as a routine practice. They suggest that parents-to-be do not critically reflect on its potential implications and lack an awareness of screening being an opt-in, rather than opt-out, procedure. During an interview, Lois (FAD midwife) claims:

> I think people have a tendency to accept what is offered to them because they think you wouldn't offer it if there wasn't a good reason to have it but they don't actually think about what can happen if they get a result they don't like. [...] With the initial booking appointment, I sometimes feel that women are coming in feeling really excited because they're pregnant and they have that first [dating] scan and most of the time, it's OK and it's all really lovely and happy. And then you go into a room and talk with them about all of the things that are not lovely and happy – HIV, syphilis, the Down's test, sickle-cell disease and thalassemia – all of these things and by the time they leave [the clinic], they often feel a bit worried and anxious and that's not the intention but it happens.

For Lois, parents-to-be accept screening on account of its accessibility but the prelude of a dating scan that ignites 'excitement' is threatened when 'you talk with them about all of the things that are not lovely and happy' such as HIV, syphilis, and Down's syndrome. The positioning of Down's syndrome with 'diseases' such as hepatitis B/C figure it as one part of the abnormal whole. If parents-to-be do truly ask midwives to 'test me for everything', as Eve suggests, Down's syndrome is cast alongside the likes of 'disease' and 'disorder', contradicting the positive imagery conjured up in the backstage accounts of professionals.

It is not too fanciful to claim that offering Down's syndrome screening in the first instance, by its very nature, categorises it in negative terms, as something worthy of early detection and potential elimination (Alderson 2001; Asch 1999; Lippman and Wilfond 1992).[13] Screening continues, according to Reynolds (2000: 894), since 'a child with Down's syndrome is seen as a disaster by many potential parents'. In the early stages of prenatal care at Freymarsh and Springtown, the condition is presented (implicitly and, in all likelihood, unintentionally) in the frontstage of the clinic in mostly negative ways. The medical work that is described here is arguably not simply a trivialisation or dismissal of the complexity of Down's syndrome (given the inconsistencies in expression rarely being vocalised) but, rather, is an important example of exclusionary practices at the mundane and implicit level, which stigmatises certain ways of being in the world (i.e. having a disability). The different prognoses for people with Down's syndrome seems to contradict the accounts of the condition in prenatal care, with the existing negative configurations arguably shaping the opinions of parents-to-be early in a pregnancy.

Once again, this analysis of categorical work is extended in Chapter 6. What is clear, for now, is that the constituting of Down's syndrome – the condition itself and its complexity and variability – is both made absent (in line with public policy) and implicitly condemned to the universal category of abnormal in prenatal care. This configuration in the medical realm exists in tension with the optimistic imaginary reflected in both empirical studies (Flaherty and Glidden 2000; Skotko 2005; Solomon 2012; Thomas 2014; Van Riper and Choi 2011; Voysey 1975) and autobiographies of parents with a child who has Down's syndrome. Focusing on the latter, mothers (e.g. Adams 2013; Clark 2008; Groneberg 2008; Lewis 2008; Soper 2009) and fathers (e.g. Austin 2014; Bérubé 1996; Daugherty 2015; Estreich 2013) have recounted their positive experiences of parenting a child with Down's syndrome. These parents recognise their situation as one which should not always be viewed as unwanted, pitiful, or tragic. Parents, indeed, often detail the happiness of raising such a child. Whilst they recognise the initial difficulties encountered when coming to terms with a diagnosis and the significant challenges (medical, social, familial, educational, vocational, political, and economic) that they face/will face on this journey, they also frame the child with Down's syndrome as a source of joy, strength, and personal growth that seems to counter dominant symbolic values around disability (Thomas 2014). This is also reflected within various forms of media – including parents' blogs and social networking websites (for more examples, see: Thomas 2015) – that ignite the formation of a 'disability public' (Ginsburg and Rapp 2015). Here, new social imaginaries of human difference become erected and people with Down's syndrome, together with their parents, are (re)constructed as occupying 'inhabitable worlds', giving them a *future* as well as a meaningful *present* (Thomas 2015).

This imaginary and formation of a Down's syndrome public is in tension with the troubled relationship that the condition has with prenatal technology. Indeed, there are two distinct 'orientations' here (Friedner 2015). For parents, documented in research and autobiographical accounts, everyday life is constituted – despite a range of clear and complicated challenges – as celebratory, life-changing (for the better), and not the disaster that it was initially believed to be. However, within the frontstage medical realm (or, at least, in Freymarsh and Springtown), where discourse shapes how people come to view and experience bodily difference, the condition is configured as a negative outcome.

Summary

In this chapter, I have identified some discrepancies regarding the constitution of Down's syndrome. In the clinic's backstage, professionals configure the condition positively, with reference to its 'compatibility with life' which is used, in turn, as a discursive resource to convey some of their personal misgivings about prenatal screening. However, Down's syndrome is rarely, if ever, discussed in frontstage consultations (nor are professionals' concerns, as highlighted in Chapter 4). Down's syndrome is made absent through its familiarity, the organisation of care, and self-professed low levels of knowledge among the necessary professionals about the condition. Absent yet present, Down's syndrome is subsequently framed within the negative collectives of 'risk', 'problem', and 'abnormality'. It is in its familiarity as something that is 'abnormal' – something one can terminate a pregnancy for – that it becomes invisible, thus preventing a discussion about the complexity and variation of the condition. So whilst Down's syndrome screening is problematically present as the topic of prenatal investigation, the condition as a state of *being* in the world is made absent, thereby accomplishing a form of bio-politics that affords the disposal and exclusion of some forms of life (Latimer and Thomas 2015).

Shakespeare (1999: 673) explains how professionals and medical texts use negative language in public rhetoric and how their clear values, implicit and subtle as they may be, reflect a consensus that 'disability is a major problem to be prevented by almost any means necessary'. Here, I capture how professionals talk this language, albeit subtly and (we assume) inadvertently, into consultations. The inconsistency in the frontstage and backstage accounts of Down's syndrome are not examples of professionals purposefully distorting information. Rather, it is an example of what people *say* or *think* they do (e.g. saying 'chance' instead of 'risk') not always translating onto the shop floor. Nonetheless, it is clear that attending to the discourses around Down's syndrome is of huge importance. For Martin (1998: 125), the very language of biological science becomes 'as real in their effects on the way doctors and patients act in the world as the effects of an antibiotic or scalpel'. This language, Martin argues, reveals some deep and powerful cultural assumptions. In Freymarsh and Springtown, the definition of Down's syndrome as a risk or abnormality, defining the identity of the future child, is produced in medical discourse and is infused with values about what a 'normal' life entails (Olarte Sierra 2010). This arguably silences cultural norms and individual values which shape understandings of certain conditions (Shakespeare 1998).

Once more, this reveals how Down's syndrome screening is entangled in 'motility' (Latimer 2007; 2013; Latimer and Munro 2006). It is this motility among professionals that accomplishes Down's syndrome, in one moment, as a condition which is compatible with life and yet, in another moment, as a risk, problem, and abnormality. Presence is, at critical moments, magnified or diminished (Strathern 1992). In Freymarsh and Springtown, positive accounts of Down's syndrome are diminished whilst discourses of risk, problem, and abnormality are magnified. It is through this motility, then, that Down's syndrome is aligned, before a diagnosis is suspected or established, with negative conceptions. I extend these arguments in Chapter 6 by describing how Down's syndrome is entwined in cultural ideologies of perfection, how mothers-to-be at an 'advanced maternal age' are implicated in this, and how the 'human' status of a foetus/baby with Down's syndrome can be *made* and *unmade* in prenatal care.

Notes

1 Independent termination statistics were not gathered at either Freymarsh or Springtown. As such, I accept that it is unfair to fully generalise extensive statistics on terminations to only two settings. However, since the termination rates have remained between 89% and 95% for over twenty years, the negative constituting of Down's syndrome in Freymarsh and Springtown suggests one plausible reason for this.

2 As will be made clear, whether Down's syndrome is 'compatible with life', or not, is not the focus of this chapter or the book. Rather, I analyse 'compatibility with life' as a discursive resource that professionals draw upon to make their claims and to account for their work and values.

3 Wilkinson (2010), a practising physician, reminds the medical profession that a small proportion of children with Edward's syndrome, a supposedly 'non-viable' condition, survive to middle or late childhood or even adulthood. Wilkinson (2010) argues that rather than question the decision to continue a pregnancy after a diagnosis of Edward's syndrome, as commonly happens, professionals should

support and engage with parents-to-be who make this tough decision. His discussion is based around a case in which a mother reports feeling abandoned and judged by professionals for continuing a pregnancy following a diagnosis of Edward's syndrome (Thiele 2010).

4 Following several conversations with parents of children with Down's syndrome, I have become aware that some of them are upset, and occasionally angered, when their child is referred to as a 'Down's baby' or 'Down's syndrome baby'. Whilst not all parents will feel this way, some are concerned that this configuration refocuses attention from the person to their condition, and that Down's syndrome should not define who their child is (instead, many parents appear to prefer the phrase 'baby/child with Down's syndrome'). However, it was clear, and worth highlighting here, that such descriptions among the professionals at Freymarsh and Springtown (more instances are cited later in this book) were not purposely designed to be malicious or insensitive.

5 Cystic fibrosis is an autosomal recessive genetic disorder that critically affects organs such as the lungs, pancreas, liver, and intestines.

6 Meetings are held monthly. A wide range of specialists gather in FMD to discuss hospital 'cases' (parents-to-be attending the clinic). Dr Karman governs proceedings and directs the gaze of attendees at a large screen displaying a list of cases. The cases are recorded in a number of ways, including whether they are under the care of Freymarsh or referred from another hospital, the condition in question, the tests already undertaken, the 'next move', the chance of survival, the outcome (death and/or delivered), and any other noteworthy contributions. The respective parents-to-be are not physically present in the meeting.

7 Various national organisations – such as the National Down Syndrome Society, the Global Down Syndrome Foundation, and the Down's Syndrome Association – have produced language/terminology guidelines to ensure that issues related to Down's syndrome are discussed in a way that is both accurate and inoffensive to the general public, including people with the condition and their families. Each organisation denounces the use of the phase 'retarded', alongside other terms, as it can be perceived as hurtful and insensitive. As with the professionals using terms such as 'Down's baby' or 'Down's syndrome baby' (see note 4), I did not perceive any nastiness from Juliana in her use of the word 'retarded'. However, this term – and this chapter as a whole – shows the importance of examining the language used when referring to Down's syndrome in prenatal care.

8 As a reminder, there are three forms of Down's syndrome: Trisomy 21 Down's syndrome (94% of cases); Mosaic Down's syndrome (2% of cases), and; Translocation Down's syndrome (4% of cases). Only Translocation Down's syndrome can be hereditary.

9 Deep vein thrombosis is the formation of blood clot in a deep vein, predominantly in the legs.

10 Rhesus disease is when antibodies in the blood of a mother-to-be destroy foetal blood cells. It only occurs when the mother-to-be has rhesus-negative blood and the father-to-be has rhesus-positive blood, leading to a diagnosis of rhesus positive blood in the foetus.

11 Sickle-cell disease is an inherited genetic blood disorder in which red blood cells develop abnormally. This affects the capacity to carry oxygen around the body.

12 Thalassemia is a form of inherited autosomal recessive blood disorder caused by the weakening and destruction of red blood cells. This affects the capacity to carry oxygen around the body.

13 According to Lippman (1991), every description of a genetic condition is a story that contains a message.

Bibliography

Adams, R. 2013. *Raising Henry: A Memoir of Motherhood, Disability, and Discovery*. New Haven, CT: Yale University Press.

Ahmed, S., Bryant, L.D., Ahmed, M., Jafri, H. and Raashid, Y. 2013. Experiences of parents with a child with Down syndrome in Pakistan and their views on termination of pregnancy. *Journal of Community Genetics* 4(1), pp. 107–114.

Alderson, P. 2001. Down's syndrome: cost, quality and value of life. *Social Science and Medicine* 53(5), pp. 627–638.

Alderson, P., Williams, C. and Farsides, B. 2004. Practitioners' views about equity within prenatal services. *Sociology* 38(1), pp. 61–80.

Armstrong, D. 1995. The rise of surveillance medicine. *Sociology of Health and Illness* 17(3), pp. 393–404.

Arribas-Ayllon, M., Sarangi, S. and Clarke, A. 2008. The micropolitics of responsibility vis-à-vis autonomy: parental accounts of childhood genetic testing and (non) disclosure. *Sociology of Health and Illness* 30(2), pp. 255–271.

Asch, A. 1999. Prenatal diagnosis and selective abortion: a challenge to practice and policy. *American Journal of Public Health* 89(11), pp. 1649–1657.

Austin, P. 2014. *Beautiful Eyes: A Father Transformed*. New York: W.W. Norton.

Bérubé, M. 1996. *Life As We Know It: A Father, a Family, and an Exceptional Child*. New York: Pantheon Books.

Boardman, F.K. 2010. *The Role of Experiential Knowledge in the Reproductive Decision Making of Families Genetically At Risk: The Case of Spinal Muscular Atrophy*. Unpublished Ph.D. Thesis, University of Warwick.

Bosk, C.L. 1992. *All God's Mistakes: Genetic Counseling in a Pediatric Hospital*. Chicago: University of Chicago Press.

Bowker, G.C. and Star, S.L. 2000. *Sorting Things Out: Classification and Its Consequences*. Cambridge, MA: MIT Press.

Bryant, L.D., Green, J.M. and Hewison, J.D. 2006. Understanding of Down's syndrome: a Q methodological investigation. *Social Science and Medicine* 63(5), pp. 1188–1200.

Bryant, L.D., Hewison, J.D. and Green, J.M. 2005. Attitudes towards prenatal diagnosis and termination in women who have a sibling with Down's syndrome. *Journal of Reproductive and Infant Psychology* 23(2), pp. 181–198.

Bryant, L.D., Murray, J., Green, J.M., Hewison, J.D., Sehmi, I. and Ellis, A. 2001. Descriptive information about Down syndrome: a content analysis of serum screening leaflets. *Prenatal Diagnosis* 21(12), pp. 1057–1063.

Burton-Jeangros, C., Cavalli, S., Gouilhers, S. and Hammer, R. 2013. Between tolerable uncertainty and unacceptable risks: how health professionals and pregnant women think about the probabilities generated by prenatal screening. *Health, Risk and Society* 15(2), pp. 144–161.

Clark, B. 2008. *A Mother Like Alex*. London: Harper True.

Clarke, A. 1994. Genetic screening: a response to Nuffield. *Bulletin of Medical Ethics* 97, 13–21.

Clarke, A.E., Shim, J.K., Mamo, L., Fosket, J.R. and Fishman, J.R. 2003. Biomedicalization: technoscientific transformations of health, illness, and US biomedicine. *American Sociological Review* 68(2), pp. 161–194.

Cleary-Goldman, J., Morgan, M.A., Malone, F.D., Robinson, J.N., Alton, M.E.D. and Schulkin, J. 2006. Screening for Down syndrome practice: patterns and knowledge of obstetricians and gynaecologists. *Obstetrics and Gynaecology* 107(1), pp. 11–17.

Cunningham-Burley, S. and Kerr, A. 1999. Defining the 'social': towards an understanding of scientific and medical discourses on the social aspects of the new human genetics. *Sociology of Health and Illness* 21(5), pp. 647–668.

Daugherty, P. 2015. *An Uncomplicated Life: A Father's Memoir of His Exceptional Daughter*. New York: HarperCollins.

Douglas, M. 1992. *Risk and Blame: Essays in Cultural Theory*. London: Routledge.

Driscoll, D.A., Morgan, M.A. and Schulkin, J. 2009. Screening for Down syndrome: changing practice of obstetricians. *American Journal of Obstetrics and Gynaecology* 200(4), pp. 459.e1–459.e9.

Ehrich, K., Williams, C. and Farsides, B. 2008. The embryo as moral work object: PGD/IVF staff views and experiences. *Sociology of Health and Illness* 30(5), pp. 772–787.

Estreich, G. 2013. *The Shape of the Eye*. New York: Tarcher Perigee.

Farrelly, E., Cho, M.K., Erby, L., Roter, D., Stenzel, A. and Ormond, K. 2012. Genetic counselling for prenatal testing: where is the discussion about disability? *Journal of Genetic Counselling* 21(6), pp. 814–824.

Flaherty, E.M. and Glidden, L.M. 2000. Positive adjustment in parents rearing children with Down syndrome. *Early Education and Development* 11(4), pp. 407–422.

Foucault, M. 1973. *The Birth of the Clinic: An Archaeology of Medical Perception*. London: Tavistock.

Foucault, M. 1979. *Discipline and Punish: The Birth of the Prison*. Harmondsworth: Penguin.

Friedner, M. 2015. *Valuing Deaf Worlds in Urban India*. New Brunswick, NJ: Rutgers University Press.

García, E., Timmermans, D.R.M. and van Leeuwen, E. 2012. Parental duties and prenatal screening: does an offer of prenatal screening lead women to believe that they are morally compelled to test? *Midwifery* 28(6), pp. 837–843.

Garfinkel, H. 1956. Conditions of successful degradation ceremonies. *American Journal of Sociology* 61(5), pp. 420–424.

Garfinkel, H. 1967. *Studies in Ethnomethodology*. Englewood Cliffs, NJ: Prentice-Hall.

Ginsburg, F. and Rapp, R. 2015. Making disability count: demography, futurity, and the making of disability publics. *Somatosphere*. Available at: http://somatosphere.net/2015/05/making-disability-count-demography-futurity-and-the-making-of-disability-publics.html [Accessed: 7 August 2016].

Goffman, E. 1971. *Relations in Public: Microstudies of the Public Order*. London: Allen Lane.

Groneberg, J.F. 2008. *Road Map to Holland: How I Found My Way Through My Son's First Two Years with Down's Syndrome*. New York: Penguin Group.

Hallowell, N. 1999. Doing the right thing: genetic risk and responsibility. *Sociology of Health and Illness* 21(5), pp. 597–621.

Helén, I. 2005. Risk management and ethics in antenatal care. In: Bunton, R. and Petersen, A. eds. *Genetic Governance: Health, Risk and Ethics in the Biotech Area*. London: Routledge, pp. 43–59.

Helm, D.T., Miranda, S. and Chedd, N.A. 1998. Prenatal diagnosis of Down syndrome: mothers' reflections on support needed from diagnosis to birth. *American Journal on Intellectual and Developmental Disabilities* 36(1), pp. 55–61.

Heyman, B., Hundy, G., Sandall, J., Spencer, K., Williams, C., Grellier, R. and Pitson, L. 2006. On being at higher risk: a qualitative study of prenatal screening for chromosomal anomalies. *Social Science and Medicine* 62(10), pp. 2360–2372.

Ivry, T. 2006. At the backstage of prenatal care: Japanese ob-gyns negotiating prenatal diagnosis. *Medical Anthropology Quarterly* 20(4), pp. 441–468.

Ivry, T. 2009. The ultrasonic picture show and the politics of threatened life. *Medical Anthropology Quarterly* 23(3), pp. 189–211.

Jones, S. 1994. *The Language of the Genes*. London: Flamingo.

Kerr, A. 2003. Governing genetics: reifying choice and progress. *New Genetics and Society* 22(2), pp. 143–158.

Kerr, A., Cunningham-Burley, S. and Amos, A. 1997. The new genetics: professionals' discursive boundaries. *The Sociological Review* 45(2), pp. 279–303.

Kerr, A., Cunningham-Burley, S. and Amos, A. 1998. Eugenics and the new genetics in Britain: examining contemporary professionals' accounts. *Science, Technology and Human Values* 23(2), 175–198.

Kevles, D. 1995. *In the Name of Eugenics. Genetics and the Uses of Human Heredity*. Cambridge, MA: Harvard University Press.

Korenromp, M.J., Page-Christiaens, G.C., van den Bout, J., Mulder, E.J. and Visser, G.H. 2007. Maternal decision to terminate pregnancy in case of Down syndrome. *American Journal of Obstetrics and Gynaecology* 196(2), pp. 149.e1–149.e11.

Latimer, J.E. 2007. Diagnosis, dysmorphology, and the family: knowledge, motility, choice. *Medical Anthropology* 26(2), pp. 97–138.

Latimer, J.E. 2013. *The Gene, the Clinic and the Family: Diagnosing Dysmorphology, Reviving Medical Dominance*. London: Routledge.

Latimer, J.E. and Munro, R. 2006. Driving the social. *The Sociological Review* 54(S1), pp. 32–53.

Latimer, J.E. and Thomas, G.M. 2015. In/exclusion in the clinic: Down's syndrome, dysmorphology, and the ethics of everyday medical work. *Sociology* 49(5), pp. 937–954.

Latour, B. 1987. *Science in Action: How to Follow Scientists and Engineers through Society*. Milton Keynes: Open University Press.

Latour, B. 1999. *Pandora's Hope: Essays on the Reality of Science Studies*. Cambridge, MA: Harvard University Press.

Lewis, S. 2008. *Living with Max*. London: Vermilion.

Lippman, A. 1991. Prenatal genetic testing and screening: constructing needs and reinforcing inequities. *American Journal of Law and Medicine* 17(1–2), pp. 15–50.

Lippman, A. and Wilfond, B.S. 1992. Twice-told tales: stories about genetic disorders. *American Journal of Human Genetics* 51(4), pp. 936–937.

Lotto, R. 2015. *Decision Making About Congenital Anomalies: How do Women and Their Partners Make the Decision to Continue or Terminate A Pregnancy Following Suspicion or Diagnosis of A Severe Congenital Anomaly?* Unpublished Ph.D. Thesis, University of Leicester.

Löwy, I. 2014. How genetics came to the unborn. *Studies in History of Philosophy of Biological and Biomedical Sciences* 47(Part A), pp. 154–162.

Lupton, D. 1999. Risk and the ontology of pregnant embodiment. In: Lupton, D. ed. *Risk and Sociocultural Theory: New Directions and Perspectives*. Cambridge: Cambridge University Press, pp. 59–85.

Lupton, D. and Tulloch, J. 2002. 'Life would be pretty dull without risk': voluntary risk-taking and its pleasures. *Health, Risk and Society* 4(2), pp. 113–124.

Madeo, A.C., Biesecker, B.B., Brasington, C., Erby, L.H. and Peters, K.F. 2011. The relationship between the genetic counselling profession and the disability community: a commentary. *American Journal of Medical Genetics Part A* 155(8), pp. 1777–1785.

Markens, S. 2013a. 'Is this something you want?' Genetic counsellors' accounts of their role in prenatal decision making. *Sociological Forum* 28(3), pp. 431–451.

Markens, S. 2013b. 'It just becomes much more complicated': genetic counsellors' views on genetics and prenatal testing. *New Genetics and Society* 32(3), pp. 302–321.

Marteau, T.M. 1995. Towards informed decisions about prenatal testing: a review. *Prenatal Diagnosis* 15(13), pp. 1215–1226.

Martin, E. 1998. The fetus as intruder: mother's bodies and medical metaphors. In: Davis-Floyd, R.E. and Dumit, J. eds. *Cyborg Babies: From Techo-Sex to Techno-Tots.* New York: Routledge, pp. 125–142.

McCourt, C. 2006. Supporting choice and control? Communication and interaction between midwives and women at the antenatal booking visit. *Social Science and Medicine* 62(6), pp. 1307–1318.

McLaughlin, J. 2003. Screening networks: shared agendas in feminist and disability movement challenges to antenatal screening and abortion. *Disability and Society* 18 (3), pp. 297–310.

Morris, J.K. and Springett, A. 2014. *The National Down Syndrome Cytogenetic Register for England and Wales: 2013 Annual Report.* London: Wolfson Institute of Preventative Medicine.

Murray, J., Cuckle, H.S., Sehmi, I., Wilson, C. and Ellis, A. 2001. Quality of written information used in Down syndrome screening. *Prenatal Diagnosis* 21(2), pp. 138–142.

NHS FASP. 2012. *NHS Fetal Anomaly Screening Programme: Annual Report 2011–2012.* University of Exeter: NHS Fetal Anomaly Screening Programme.

Olarte Sierra, M.F. 2010. *Achieving the Desirable Nation: Abortion and Antenatal Testing in Colombia (the Case of Amniocentesis).* Unpublished Ph.D. Thesis, University of Amsterdam.

Pascale, C.M. 2011. *Cartographies of Knowledge: Exploring Qualitative Epistemologies.* London: Sage.

Pilnick, A. 2008. 'It's something for you both to think about': choice and decision-making in nuchal translucency screening for Down's syndrome. *Sociology of Health and Illness* 30(4), pp. 511–530.

Possamai-Inesedy, A. 2006. Confining risk: choice and responsibility in childbirth within a risk society. *Health Sociology Review* 15(4), pp. 406–414.

Press, N. and Browner, C.H. 1997. Why women say yes to prenatal diagnosis. *Social Science and Medicine* 45(7), pp. 979–989.

Rapp, R. 1988. Chromosomes and communication: the discourse of genetic counseling. *Medical Anthropology Quarterly* 2(2), pp. 143–157.

Rapp, R. 2000. *Testing Women, Testing the Fetus: The Social Impact of Amniocentesis in America.* London: Routledge.

Rappert, B. and Bauchspies, W.K. 2014. Introducing absence. *Social Epistemology: A Journal of Knowledge, Culture and Policy* 28(1): 1–3.

Reist, M.T. 2006. *Defiant Birth: Women Who Resist Medical Eugenics.* North Melbourne, VIC: Spinifex Press.

Reynolds, T. 2000. Down's syndrome screening: a controversial test, with more controversy to come! *Journal of Clinical Pathology* 53(12), pp. 893–898.

Rothman, B.K. 1986. *The Tentative Pregnancy: Amniocentesis and the Sexual Politics of Motherhood*. London: Pandora.

Saxton, M. 2013. Disability rights and selective abortion. In: Davis, L.J. ed. *The Disability Studies Reader*. 3rd edn. London: Routledge, pp. 120–132.

Scamell, M. and Alaszewski, A. 2012. Fateful moments and the categorisation of risk: midwifery practice and the ever-narrowing window of normality during childbirth. *Health, Risk and Society* 14(2), pp. 207–221.

Shakespeare, T.W. 1995. Disabled people and the new genetics. *Genethics News* 5, pp. 8–11.

Shakespeare, T.W. 1998. Choices and rights: eugenics, genetics and disability equality. *Disability and Society* 13(5), pp. 665–681.

Shakespeare, T.W. 1999. 'Losing the plot'? Medical and activist discourses of contemporary genetics and disability. *Sociology of Health and Illness* 21(5), pp. 669–688.

Shakespeare, T.W. 2006. *Disability Rights and Wrongs*. London: Routledge.

Skirton, H. and Barr, O. 2007. Influences on uptake of antenatal screening for Down's syndrome: a review of the literature. *Evidence Based Midwifery* 5(1), pp. 4–9.

Skirton, H. and Barr, O. 2010. Antenatal screening and informed choice: a cross-sectional survey of parents and professionals. *Midwifery* 26(6), pp. 596–602.

Skotko, B.G. 2005. Prenatally diagnosed Down syndrome: mothers who continued their pregnancies evaluate their health care providers. *American Journal of Obstetrics and Gynaecology* 192(3), pp. 670–677.

Solomon, A. 2012. *Far From the Tree: Parents, Children and the Search for Identity*. London: Vintage.

Soper, K.L. 2009. *Gifts: Mothers Reflect on How Children with Down Syndrome Enrich Their Lives*. Bethesda, MA: Woodbine House.

Strathern, M. 1992. *Reproducing the Future: Anthropology, Kinship, and the New Reproductive Technologies*. New York: Routledge.

Taussig, M. 1999. *Defacement: Public Secrecy and the Labor of the Negative*. Stanford, CA: Stanford University Press.

Ternby, E., Ingvoldstad, C., Annerén, G. and Axelsson, O. 2015a. Midwives and information on prenatal testing with focus on Down syndrome. *Prenatal Diagnosis* 35(12), pp. 1202–1207.

Ternby, E., Ingvoldstad, C., Annerén, G., Lindgren, P. and Axelsson, O. 2015b. Information and knowledge about Down syndrome among women and partners after first trimester combined testing. *Acta Obstetrica et Gynaecologica Scandinavica* 94(3), pp. 329–332.

Thiele, P. 2010. He was my son, not a dying baby. *Journal of Medical Ethics* 36(11), pp. 646–647.

Thomas, G.M. 2014. Cooling the mother out: revisiting and revising Goffman's account. *Symbolic Interaction* 37(2), pp. 283–299.

Thomas, G.M. 2015. Un/inhabitable worlds: the curious case of Down's syndrome. *Somatosphere*. Weblog [Online]. 29 August. Available at: http://somatosphere.net/2015/07/uninhabitable-worlds-the-curious-case-of-downs-syndrome.html [Accessed: 7 August 2016].

Thomas, G.M. 2016. An elephant in the consultation room? Configuring Down syndrome in UK antenatal care. *Medical Anthropology Quarterly* 30(2), pp. 238–258.

Thomas, G.M. and Rothman, B.K. 2016. Keeping the backdoor to eugenics ajar? Disability and the future of prenatal screening. *American Medical Association Journal of Ethics* 18(4), pp. 406–415.

Tymstra, T., Bosboom, J. and Bouman, K. 2004. Prenatal diagnosis of Down's syndrome: experiences of women who decided to continue the pregnancy. *International Journal of Risk and Safety in Medicine* 16(2), pp. 91–96.

Van Riper, M. and Choi, H. 2011. Family–provider interactions surrounding the diagnosis of Down syndrome. *Genetics in Medicine* 13(8), pp. 714–716.

Voysey, M. 1975. *A Constant Burden: The Reconstitution of Family Life*. London: Routledge and Kegan Paul.

Wilkinson, D.J.C. 2010. Antenatal diagnosis of trisomy 18, harm and parental choice. *Journal of Medical Ethics* 36(11), pp. 644–645.

Williams, C., Alderson, P. and Farsides, B. 2002a. 'Drawing the line' in prenatal screening and testing: health practitioners' discussions. *Health, Risk and Society* 4(1), pp. 61–75.

Williams, C., Alderson, P. and Farsides, B. 2002b. Is nondirectiveness possible within the context of antenatal screening and testing? *Social Science and Medicine* 54(3), pp. 339–347.

Williams, C., Alderson, P. and Farsides, B. 2002c. What constitutes 'balanced' information in the practitioners' portrayal of Down's syndrome? *Midwifery* 18(3), pp. 230–237.

Chapter 6

Expectant parents, expecting perfection

Extending the arguments of Chapter 5, I begin this chapter by exploring how constitutions of Down's syndrome in negative terms connect with cultural ideologies around 'ab/normality' and 'im/perfection' that emerge via social practices (mostly NT scans) and cultural materials. These positionings are primarily established in the early stages of prenatal care. Whilst professionals worry that parents-to-be have rather unrealistic expectations about pregnancy and infant health, they simultaneously reinforce their lay beliefs (particularly around 'normality' and 'perfection') and, in so doing, figure Down's syndrome – before a diagnosis is suspected or established – as disrupting expectations and as a deviation in the embodiment of prenatal expectation. This emphasis on normality and perfection also institutes mothers-to-be, primarily, as responsible for promising flawlessness in a foetus/baby. Confronted with endless reminders of 'perfect baby' outcomes, I capture how mothers, and particularly mothers aged thirty-five or above (using medical discourse, at an 'advanced maternal age'), are disciplined into considering pregnancy as pathological and, potentially, screening for Down's syndrome as one means through which they assure a 'perfect' outcome.

Finally, I identify how constitutions of Down's syndrome and cultural ideals of 'normality' are enacted by discursive shifts in FMD between 'foetus' and 'baby' once a diagnosis of Down's syndrome is established or largely suspected. Whilst ultrasound scans and/or foetal movement often gives rise to a foetus *becoming* a baby, the identification of a suspected diagnosis can involve re-figuring the baby as, once more, a foetus. This shift not only allows professionals to accomplish emotional and moral distance from the issues at hand but also highlights the malleability of the human category whilst transforming particular entities – including a foetus with Down's syndrome – into something potentially disposable. This classificatory work restores order and re-establishes boundaries in the clinic, particularly between 'normal' and 'abnormal', that is integral to the routine functioning of prenatal care. To conclude, I argue that a combination of all of these elements, bringing ideals of what is 'normal' and 'perfect' close to hand, positions both parents and the born/unborn child with Down's syndrome in certain ways.

In this chapter, there will be no engagement with moral arguments around termination, such as whether terminating for Down's syndrome should be classified as acceptable or not. Here, I agree with the stance of McLaughlin (2003) who suggests that analyses of screening should not prioritise the rights and wrongs of terminating a foetus but, rather, should examine both the social values and structural inequalities which promote this choice and which discriminate against disabled people (more on this in Chapter 7). This chapter, in essence, unpacks the conditions under which a termination for the condition is made possible. In so doing, it shows, with Shakespeare (2000), that deliberations on this matter should be more nuanced than simplistic 'pro-life versus pro-choice' or 'eugenics versus choice' arguments.

Producing perfection

In Chapter 5, I described how discourses (risk, problem, abnormality) sustain a negative constitution of Down's syndrome. These are commonly created and reinforced through the opposing and interweaving discourses of 'normal' and 'perfect'. What constitutes normality and perfection is built into everyday language, particularly assumptions around how we organise particular bodies. The dualism of 'normal' and 'abnormal' is formally demarcated after twenty-four weeks of a pregnancy during which parents-to-be can access a legal termination due to, in the words of FMD, 'medical problems'. However, as recognised in Chapter 2, a termination is a grey area owing to a lack of specificity in the Abortion Act 1967 about what pregnancies can be categorised as 'viable' or 'non-viable' (HM Government 2016). Whilst a precise definition of what constitutes a serious 'medical problem' is difficult, its interpretation is not. Indeed, what is viewed as normal or abnormal is accomplished in the early stages of prenatal care before a diagnosis is suspected or established. In the following extract taken from an NT scan, Sophie (SAD sonographer) describes the procedure to Mr and Mrs Reed (parents-to-be):

> SOPHIE: Did you have the NT scan with your previous child?
> MRS REED: No. I've had it now because I'm a bit worried with being quite a bit older.
> SOPHIE: OK. [Sophie moves the transducer across the abdomen] There's the baby's head [pointing]. Baby is nice and flat here. And that's a nice and small NT.
> MRS REED: Great.
> SOPHIE: [Nuchal translucency measures at 1.56mm]. We're all fine here. It's actually one of the clearest scans I've seen. That's perfect that is. Baby is lying perfectly on its back. [...] That's all looking very normal and lovely. The NT is 1.5mm and we want it below 3mm so that's very good. The actual measurement is 1.56mm. So there's the little arm there, the hand there too.

MRS REED: There's a history of anencephaly[1] in my family so could you check for that as well please?

SOPHIE: Yes OK. [Mrs Reed turns to the monitor] That seems fine to me.

MRS REED: Good. It's just there are three cases in my Mum's family. There's a history of spina bifida[2] and anencephaly.

SOPHIE: [Looks back at Mrs Reed] That's a very, very normal looking baby to me. I would normally be able to see anencephaly. It is a very obvious abnormality. It all looks fine. I can't check for spina bifida though because it's too soon. It's a healthy looking baby there.

After Mrs Reed accounts for her decision-making by citing the worry stemming from her 'being quite a bit older' than in her previous pregnancy, Sophie describes the baby's (not foetus') attributes, specifically the neck fluid, as 'nice and small', as 'perfect', and as 'looking very normal and lovely'. Sophie validates her contentions by referring to a measurement of 1.56mm as 'very good' since it falls under 3mm. Sophie then constructs other features of the baby as 'normal', with Mrs Reed seeking confirmation of this owing to a family history of other 'cases', albeit not Down's syndrome. Sophie responds by telling Mrs Reed that she is carrying a 'healthy' and 'very, very normal looking baby'. Whilst Sophie discounts the 'obvious abnormality' of anencephaly, the perceived absence of markers for Down's syndrome and any other 'abnormality' means that the baby is perceived as 'normal'. Since sonographers only detect markers for a condition rather than a concrete diagnosis only available via diagnostic testing, they rely on the provisional absence of indicators as a likely sign of a disability-free outcome. Much like in FAD, Down's syndrome, here, is categorised alongside other conditions (anencephaly and spina bifida) as an 'abnormality'. Prenatal technologies, thus, become apparatuses through which a foetus is categorised as normal/abnormal and perfect/imperfect.

The close monitoring of both mothers-to-be and foetuses, together with standards of 'normality' imposed by and governing obstetrics, resonate with an idea of perfect, or at least desirable, people/future people (Olarte Sierra 2010). Feminist and disability scholars have critiqued the role of prenatal technologies in fostering expectations of giving birth to 'perfect' children (Rapp 2000; Remennick 2006; Rothman 1986). But if technology is perceived as a resource that 'promises to produce the perfect child' (Landsman 1998: 77) and ensures that a baby is healthy (Remennick 2006), one should ask what this category of perfection entails. If the perfect child represents an object of cultural desire, we must contextualise it to a particular society or institution. Buchbinder and Timmermans (2012: 61) suggest that perfection, despite its 'implied universality and normative power', is a 'deeply contextual concept contingent on its cultural and historical framing'. Although Rapp (2000) and Buchbinder and Timmermans (2012) identify the quest for baby perfection as distinctly American, such an expedition is certainly not confined to US waters.

In Freymarsh and Springtown, the pursuit of perfection/normality (the terms are used interchangeably hereafter) is accomplished in the social practices of the prenatal clinic, and particularly in NT scans. Since parents-to-be commonly struggle to establish the physiological structure of foetuses during an ultrasound scan, the sonographer – as 'host' or 'tourist guide' – strategically performs and transforms the chaotic image into a 'baby' and parents-to-be into families (Krol økke 2011: 22). During an NT scan, Sophie (SAD sonographer) describes what she sees on the monitor to Mr and Mrs Stock (parents-to-be):

SOPHIE: You see these white lines here on the monitor [points]? We measure between those and that's the nuchal translucency. We like them under 3mm. It's 1.26mm on first measurement, which is fine.

MRS STOCK: That's around the same as it was during the previous pregnancy. It was pretty small.

SOPHIE: Yes, perfect. It's nice and small, which is great. Based on the scan alone, that's a very low-risk [Mr and Mrs Stock smile].
[...]

SOPHIE: [Sophie prints pictures of the imaging] These pictures look absolutely fine scan wise. It all looks good. All fabulous.

MRS STOCK: Good.

MR STOCK: Great.

SOPHIE: There we go [Sophie gives the pictures to Mr Stock]. It looks more human now. They move all over the place! [Mr and Mrs Stock laugh. Sophie continues the scan] Here you are: a beautiful baby.

MRS STOCK: Oh let's have a look then! [Takes picture from Mr Stock] It's a baby!

MR STOCK: How's the size of the baby?

SOPHIE: The size is fine and normal.
[...]

MRS STOCK: I was having it just for peace of mind really. I'm thirty-eight.

SOPHIE: Well you've got a perfect baby so you've got nothing to worry about! Yours is a nice and small one. I can see the one in your last pregnancy was 1.02mm which is really small. The smallest I've ever seen here is 0.98mm.

Sophie describes the 'baby' as 'perfect' with a 'nice and small' measurement which, according to Sophie, points toward a 'very low-risk'. A perfect baby corresponds to imagining lower-risk futures. Reassuring utterances of 'it all looks good' and 'all fabulous' collude to shape expectations of perfection and of a 'beautiful baby', with Sophie joking that the baby 'looks more human now' since movement can obscure image quality. Ultrasound provides an ample opportunity for revitalising expectations among parents-to-be and for relieving any anxiety, particularly in the case of Mrs Stock, who accounts for her reason to undertake screening ('I'm thirty-eight'). Sophie reduces her angst by shaping her understanding of the nuchal translucency as 'nice and small' with reference to her experiential knowledge ('the smallest I've seen here is 0.98').

During NT scans, producing perfection emerges not only through the reassuring utterances of 'normal' and 'perfect' but also through the sonographer and parents-to-be engaging in a process of 'collaborative coding' which becomes essential to making the imagery on the screen personally and socially meaningful (Roberts 2012). Here, the physiological attributes of the foetus become markers of perfection. Ultrasound scans create an encounter in which participants can distinguish the foetus as a consumable 'baby' and can offer opportunities for gendered and 'good' parental performances, for constructing familial relations, and for gazing at the 'perfect' child (Gammeltoft 2007; Kr.løkke 2011; Müller-Rockstroh 2011; Roberts 2012; Taylor 2008). Perfect/normal babies, as a culturally contingent category, have desirable physiological traits such as 'cute toes', 'little hands', 'Buddha bellies', 'button noses', and 'big beautiful eyes' among others. In addition, they 'perform' when the camera rolls, with their movement being playfully attributed to being 'active', 'cheeky', and/or 'naughty'. This contributes to creating and sustaining cultural ideologies of normality – and, so, also abnormality – in a baby.

This notion of normality/perfection is accomplished further in the materiality of the clinic, particularly Springtown. As a privately funded company, there is greater freedom – in comparison to Freymarsh – to encourage consumption and pursue monetary profit through selling pregnancy goods (more on this later in the chapter). Freymarsh, in contrast, was not allowed to offer commercially available goods, nor was it permitted to adorn walls with photographs of its own choosing. However, the hospital still organises pregnancy around discourses of perfection, via materials including prenatal literature and media tendering 'advice' to mothers-to-be. In short, in both Freymarsh and Springtown, the pathways and flows constituting the building's physicality are symbolic in relation to the pursuit of normality/perfection during a pregnancy. After every NT scan in Freymarsh and Springtown, for instance, parents-to-be are tendered a picture of their baby. Obtaining a picture is a key moment in the pregnancy ritual. Producing such materials not only helps construct and maintain identities (Taylor 2008) but also accomplishes ideas around the perfect baby. The following fieldnotes taken at SAD describe the clinic's space, the first passage taken from the first day of fieldwork and the second passage taken from around five months into the study:

> Pictures of unborn and newborn babies are plastered around the clinic. [...] Lisa [sonographer] takes me into the room where ultrasound scans are performed. The room is approximately 4×4 metres with only four to five people able to comfortably occupy the space. The room is dark and

contains three chairs, a trolley, a computer, and an ultrasound machine. The room's walls are adorned with two images of 'water babies'.[3]

A '5D-photo stand' greets me as I enter the clinic. I have not seen this before. The products on display are 3D-photo-laser engraved crystal glass objects, in a variety of shapes and sizes, depicting images of unborn babies, newborn babies, families, and a dog.

With its walls adorned with images of newborn/unborn babies (e.g. 'water babies') and its offers of purchasable keepsakes to memorialise the unborn (e.g. '5D-photo stand'), SAD accomplishes ideals not only around the perfect baby but also around the 'normal' future family. The combination of cultural materials and social practices in producing perfection is accentuated in the commercial availability of '4D baby-bonding' ultrasound scans which are performed around twenty-four to thirty-two weeks into a pregnancy. In SAD, 4D scans are advertised as promoting maternal 'bonding', as providing reassurance, and as tendering entertaining experiences for parents-to-be (Thomas 2015). The scans provide detailed real-time images of a foetus and often culminate in the production of detailed photographs and 'keepsake DVDs' (Gammeltoft 2007). In one flyer, Springtown describes the 4D scan as:

[Producing] lifelike images like a moving statue allowing parents to clearly see their baby smile, yawn, blink or swallow etc. as they move inside their secret world.

The 'baby' is categorised as a smiling, yawning, and blinking 'moving statue'. In other artefacts distributed by Springtown, parents-to-be are told that they will see 'their unborn child at play', receive a 'twenty minute video recording on a keepsake DVD and four to six colour photographs', and that 'bonding between parents and baby has been shown to be stronger when the 3D image is seen compared to the 2D image because the picture of the baby is more realistic'. Such materials, in unison with interactional exchanges in the scan room, not only transform the prenatal clinic into a site of consumption but also organise the expected conduct of mothers-to-be – who can experience the benefit of 'bonding' from the scan[4] – and figures the baby as a consumable entity.

But how does this relate specifically to Down's syndrome? By blurring the boundary between medicine and consumption, I suggest that the 4D scan – alongside other ultrasound scans – and the materials of the clinic contribute to changing an anticipation of a normal child into a normative expectation. Such playful practices in the ultrasound room, whilst carefully designed to provide an entertaining and pleasant experience for parents-to-be, construct the ideal (perfect) body and the ideal family that are based on problematic cultural ideals, thus shaping bodies and families in ways which may not correlate with future outcomes. Any deviation from the imagined child, therefore, is viewed as an undesirable outcome. When discussing the idea of prenatal perfection during an interview, Esther (SAD sonographer) claims:

> We want everything to be perfect and it's not. It's about having compassion for things that aren't necessarily perfect. [...] My experience has shown me that once women are told there's an anomaly, whether it's an isolated cleft lip or club foot, the baby is no longer perfect. The women's imagination is often a million times worse than the real thing.

Esther highlights how any 'anomaly', regardless of prognosis, makes a baby 'no longer perfect' since the image conjured up in the imagination of mothers-to-be is 'often a million times worse than the real thing'. Martha (FAD midwife) similarly claims, during an interview, that when mothers-to-be receive a higher-risk result, this means that 'the fact that they're high-risk and their baby might not be perfect is all that they can see'. In one conversation, Gail (FAD midwife) explains:

> The public don't like the thought of something that's not perfect. We want everything to be perfect. It's like we can't have anybody who's handicapped or not quite perfect. It's quite sad then when you do have a baby with Down's syndrome because of the way our culture is. It's like shameful isn't it? Like, this baby's not perfect, but it's just life really isn't it?

Gail suggests that 'our culture', referring to an abstract UK culture rather than medical culture, demarcates Down's syndrome as 'shameful' and 'not perfect'. In Chapter 5, I highlighted the view of professionals that Down's syndrome is familiar to parents-to-be because of its 'face' (Latimer 2013), that is, the distinctive anatomical features of people with the condition. This, arguably, also constitutes a reason why Down's syndrome is seen as non-perfect. During a conversation with Dominique and Hannah (administrative staff) in the Springtown office (as a reminder, administrative staff in the office book NT scans for parents-to-be), Dominique identifies the popularity of NT scans over cardiac scans because people are 'more frightened of Down's syndrome kids, the costs and that', whilst Hannah suggests that the 'visible thing' of Down's syndrome is not wanted by parents. Cardiac defects, however, are not immediately visual and so, she concludes, 'the child becomes normal'. Here, the 'face' of Down's syndrome is enacted as a metonym for abnormality and imperfection more generally.

In a previous study, I described how feelings of 'sadness', 'grief', 'sickness', 'fear', 'failure', 'blame', 'anger' and 'devastation' were expressed by mothers when discussing initial reactions to their child's diagnosis of Down's syndrome (Thomas 2014: 5). This often corresponds to mothers initially conceiving of their child as a 'monster'; '[i]t is only because, as human beings, we are living beings, that a morphological defect is, to our living eyes, a monster' (Canguilhem 2005: 187). For many mothers, the physical markers of Down's syndrome, as a 'discredited stigma' (Goffman 1963: 49), initially contributed to feelings of 'alien kinship' since the child disrupted normative maternal/familial expectations and threatened their presentation of family normality (Rapp 1995: 81). One might suspect that the imagined 'face' of Down's syndrome is an imperfect deviation in the embodiment of expectation (Rothman 1998; Rapp 2000) and, as such, children with Down's syndrome are viewed as 'impaired, imperfect, damaged goods, unsatisfactory merchandise on the commodity exchange of conventional kid culture' (Rapp 1999: xiii). It is worth noting, too, that having a disabled child may also 'transform' motherhood by giving parents 'the gift of their own self-knowledge' (1999: xiii). Yet this positive configuration, as shown in Chapter 5, is often absent in prenatal consultations.

Perfection and older mothers: 'elderly primigravidas'

So how does this image of ab/normality – built into the interactions and materiality of FAD and SAD – figure mothers-to-be and fathers-to-be? In Chapter 4, it was claimed that screening implicates parents-to-be, though mothers-to-be more than fathers-to-be,[5] in relation to decision-making processes. Equally, mothers-to-be and especially those at an 'advanced maternal age', clinically defined, are directly implicated in cultural ideologies around perfection in pregnancy. An increased maternal age, translating to women aged thirty-five and above, is the only known attribute that increases the chance of a Down's syndrome diagnosis (see: Chapter 2). The discourse of 'advanced maternal age', reinforced through the production of these risk factors, positions mothers-to-be aged thirty-five plus at an increased risk of having a child with Down's syndrome. This is illustrated in the following fieldnotes taken during an NT scan between Sophie (SAD sonographer) and Mrs Fallon (mother-to-be):

> SOPHIE: That's the nasal bone [points]. It's often absent in babies with Down's syndrome so that's good.
> MRS FALLON: OK. I'm forty-two now so ...
> SOPHIE: It's depressing when you read the literature isn't it?
> MRS FALLON: Yes. I know I'm a one in sixty-five risk on my age alone. That's the trouble when you put off having another baby.

Mrs Fallon's age and risk status appear to be used to account for her decision to undertake an NT scan. Unlike Mrs Fallon, many mothers-to-be in Freymarsh and Springtown do not appear to know their standalone risk factor but, rather, do have a vague awareness of older mothers-to-be being more susceptible to a Down's syndrome diagnosis. For instance, Miranda (mother-to-be) justifies her decision to undertake a NT scan rather than quadruple screening (the former is more accurate than the latter) by asserting 'I had the blood test the last time I was pregnant but I'm older now so I got a bit worried'. Risk discourse brings out social accounting practices in particularly forceful ways (Horlick-Jones 2005); it becomes a 'forensic resource [...] a language with which to hold persons accountable' (Douglas 1992: 22). During an interview, Lisa (SAD sonographer) explains why older mothers-to-be attend Springtown rather than an NHS hospital:

> The older you are, the more likely you are to have had more pregnancies with problems in. There's a perception that being an older mother brings with it medical problems as well so older women want a bit more tender-loving-care than they'd get in the NHS. I think someone early on in the pregnancy tells them 'you're an elderly primigravida' [laughs] when you're a certain age and you think 'God, really?' And then you realise you're suddenly categorised as higher-risk.

Lisa says that older mothers-to-be are more likely to experience 'medical problems', meaning that they often account for their attendance at Springtown with reference to their age. By light-heartedly citing the term 'elderly primigravida', defined as a woman pregnant with her first child after the age of thirty-five (*primus* being Latin for first and *gravidus* meaning pregnant), Lisa highlights how older mothers-to-be are 'categorised as higher-risk' in prenatal care. Armed with this risk knowledge, mothers-to-be may reconstruct their identity to being someone susceptible to having a baby with Down's syndrome. Possamai-Inesedy (2006) claims that women respond as if risk, as a concrete entity, actually exists; risks become actualised through anticipation and call for a person to respond. In the context of Down's syndrome screening, this response can involve undertaking a more accurate procedure, namely mothers-to-be aged over thirty-five having an NT scan at SAD rather than a quadruple screen at FAD. Mothers-to-be accounting for their decision to opt for screening by citing their age arguably points to the procedure as just one more component of their regimes of ritual purity along with 'lifestyle choices' (diet, taking folic acid, avoiding certain activities, and so on). Such rituals are enacted as part of, as Martha (FAD midwife) claims, their 'quest for the perfect child'. Other research recognises, indeed, that parents-to-be consent to screening as part of their pursuit of perfection, that is, by wanting to acquire reassurance that their baby is healthy and disability-free (Lupton 2013; Olarte Sierra 2010; Remennick 2006).

The configuration of older mothers as at-risk is exemplified further in the following fieldnotes taken in a screening consultation between Toni (FAD midwife) and Mrs Hooper (mother-to-be):

> TONI: Have you thought about whether you want screening and testing?
> MRS HOOPER: To be honest, when I was offered screening, I just said yes for everything. But now I know about [the possibility of miscarrying

after amniocentesis], I'll probably not have the amniocentesis but I
want to know about the risk factor.

TONI: So you're having the screening for informational purposes?

MRS HOOPER: Yes.

TONI: That's fine. To be fair, you're a good age anyway. When you get
older, your risk of having a baby with Down's syndrome increases.
When you get to thirty-five, it all goes downhill and when you get
to forty, it goes *really* downhill!

Toni smirks as Mrs Hooper appears to smile uncomfortably.

Here, Toni reassures Mrs Hooper by classifying her as a 'good age' and
those aged thirty-five and above as 'going downhill', that is, a bad age. Here,
the older mother-to-be is figured as problematic, an at-risk figure who may be
subtly coerced into undertaking medical intervention via diagnostic testing.
In her work on paediatric and genetic medicine, Dimond (2013) claims that
the category of patient is 'fuzzy', extending to implicate a number of people
including children, parents, and family members. Likewise, in Freymarsh and
Springtown, a mother-to-be and foetus are frequently reduced to a single
entity. In this metonymical move, mothers-to-be are ascribed the provisional
status of higher-risk/lower-risk (Mrs Fallon: 'I was a 1 in 65 risk'). Consider
the following quotes taken from professionals during their interactions with
parents-to-be (and that have already been cited in this book): 'you'll be placed
in either the lower-risk or higher-risk bracket and if you're higher-risk, you're
advised to have an amniocentesis'; 'the older you are, the higher your risk is for
having a baby with Down's syndrome'; 'what I badly need to know is whether
you want to know whether you're a lower-risk or higher-risk'. Mothers-to-be,
thus, receive *their* risk; *they* are the ones at-risk in screening practices.

With screening colonised by a risk discourse and both the mother-to-be
and foetus being classified as a single entity, it is feasible that older
mothers-to-be may feel anxiety and self-blame should expectations be brea-
ched (i.e. if receiving a higher-risk result and/or diagnosis). This depiction
has been perpetuated by the media, with prevailing visual representations of
pregnant women excluding the pregnant body of the older mother (Budds
et al. 2013). It is illuminated further in Springtown through offering
mothers-to-be 'Body Clock Testing', a procedure which makes it possible,
according to the advertising leaflet, 'to predict future fertility'. The leaflet urges
women, and specifically women 'leaving it late', to 'take control of their
reproductive choices' by undertaking a test which can cure 'the unknown'
by '[taking] out the uncertainty' which will help women to 'understand her
choices'. It reads:

More and more women leave it until later to try for a pregnancy with
nearly 20% of women leaving it until after 35 to start a family. Many

however find that they have left it too late, even with help from treatments like IVF. A woman's natural conception rate falls from about 20% a cycle at 30 years old to 5% a cycle at 40. Although high profile celebrities like Amy Ryan, Madonna, Celine Dion and Halle Berry have had much publicised pregnancies in their late 30s and 40s, women's biological body clocks have not changed and for many it may be too late! The test has been developed amidst warnings of complacency from leading UK fertility experts. Couples are 'sticking their heads in the sand' and one expert urged all 30-year-old women to take a 'fertility MOT' test.

After supposedly certifying their claims with reference to scientific knowledge, celebrities, and 'leading UK fertility experts', women are accused of 'complacency' and 'sticking their heads in the sand' in relation to reproductive decision-making. The leaflet draws on claims made by Professor Bill Ledger, who urges all thirty-year-old women to 'take a "fertility MOT" test' since 'Britain is facing a fertility timebomb' (Hill and Asthana 2009). The urging and disciplining of women to take this particular test is epitomised by the picture accompanying the text: a woman sleeping and holding an alarm clock whilst facing the reader.

The social practices (e.g. consultations) and cultural materials (e.g. leaflets) of Freymarsh and Springtown constitute the categorisation of 'at-risk' older mothers who, at an 'advanced maternal age', are accountable for their conduct. Whilst the vast majority of prenatal literature and policy urges choice and autonomy, these discourses are problematic once highlighted alongside the alleged risks prevailing with an advancing maternal age (Budds et al. 2013). This illuminates the dominant ideologies of motherhood prevailing in our risk culture whereby mothers are constantly (re)positioned and where children become expressions and extensions of the maternal self. In an era of 'total motherhood' (Wolf 2011: 71), mothers must detect and eradicate every 'risk' to their child regardless of personal cost. Moral codes discipline mothers-to-be into viewing risks as calculable and preventable, urging them to be reflexively vigilant about their bodies, even before conception, in anticipation of pregnancy and motherhood. In the waiting room of FAD, for example, two televisions show BabyTV on repeat (BabyTV is also explained in Chapter 1). Advertised as an information channel with the tagline 'keeping you informed', it offers parents-to-be advice on concerns such as appropriate cots, breastfeeding, and car safety. This depicts parenthood as something to be managed and disciplined into, a pedagogic accomplishment containing (moral) statements about the appropriate conduct of the 'good parent'. The subtle coercion of mothers-to-be into particular patterns of conduct reflects a form of pastoral power (Foucault 1979), whereby any deviation from what is seen as 'normal' is framed as irresponsible.

In the context of Down's syndrome screening, the practice is likely to be perceived as the expected and responsible action for those at an 'advanced maternal age'; to not engage in risk-avoiding conduct could be considered as 'a failure of the self to take care of itself – a form of irrationality' (Greco 1993: 361). It seems that responsible (future) parenting implies the acquisition of all available medical information about the health of a foetus (García et al. 2012) and submitting to biomedical surveillance to potentially produce a 'normal' baby (Gottfreðsdóttir et al. 2009). Since women tend to be held responsible for child care and family welfare, and as normative expectations concerning familial formation hold considerable power in many societies, 'anxieties regarding reproductive outcomes often run deep' (Gammeltoft and Wahlberg 2014: 211). This can explain why some mothers-to-be, responsible for ensuring a perfect outcome, can experience feelings of culpability and blame if this expectation is not realised (Alderson 2001; Buchbinder and Timmermans 2012; García et al. 2012; Gross 2010; Ivry 2006; Landsman 2009; Latimer 2007; Rapp 2000; Reed 2012; Remennick 2006; Thomas 2014; Thomas and Lupton 2016). This is grounded in an idea that a foetus/baby is neither inherently perfect nor imperfect but, rather, is 'a perfectible creature' (Ivry 2006: 459). In other words, the outcome of a foetus is framed as the product of diligent mothers-to-be rather than being a random assemblage of genes and chromosomes. Screening for Down's syndrome, as such, is arguably viewed as an important type of care-work that is integral to assuming the role of a 'good mother'. Located in powerful cultural discourses related to good parenthood, screening instigates a process in which mothers-to-be become 'patients-in-waiting' (Timmermans and Buchbinder 2010: 408) and, should further testing be required, re-enter a site in which genetic knowledge becomes 'actionable' (Timmermans and Shostak 2016: 44). The point here is that, by promoting the 'normality' of a foetus, and mothers-to-be being solely responsible for this, Down's syndrome screening becomes an obligatory passage point on the road to parenthood, thus further routinising the procedure in prenatal care. We can ask, then, whether these choices are viewed, in fact, as compulsions.

Making and unmaking the foetus/baby

Extending the attention on how ideas of normality are accomplished in the social and material life of both Freymarsh and Springtown, the remainder of this chapter explores how a possible pregnancy termination is discussed within Down's syndrome screening consultations and other encounters pre-dominantly taking place in FMD. This begins by citing a conversation between Nicola (FAD midwife) and Mrs Li (mother-to-be) from a Down's syndrome screening consultation:

NICOLA: I'm going to tell you about the test and then I'm going to take you through so you can have your bloods done. So you're offered the screening test today. It won't tell you if the baby has Down's syndrome but it provides a risk ratio which gives a lower-risk or higher-risk of the condition. If you're a higher-risk, we telephone you within three to five working days where you're invited back here. You'll receive counselling and you're offered a further diagnostic test called an amniocentesis. Have you heard of it?

MRS LI: Yes. I had one in the last pregnancy. Actually, I'm going back to Cambodia in a few days for three weeks. What can we do? I'm back on [date] when I'm having the [anomaly] scan.

NICOLA: Well the amniocentesis should take place in three and a half weeks because if you wanted to terminate, it's leaving it very late in the pregnancy. [Mrs Li looks concerned] If you came back as higher-risk, would you have an amniocentesis? Because if not, you might have to think whether having this test would be the best option. You could be higher-risk but it could all still be OK.

MRS LI: I would rather know if I was higher-risk.

NICOLA: OK. Well if you ring in six days' time, we might have your result. If you're higher-risk, we can book you an amniocentesis over the phone. But you should really consider this because obviously the baby will be at such an advanced gestation for amniocentesis and potentially a termination.

MRS LI: I understand.

NICOLA: How old are you?

MRS LI: Thirty-three.

NICOLA: OK. If you did want an amniocentesis, you would be counselled beforehand. It has a 1% risk of miscarriage and if there's a diagnosis, you're offered a termination of pregnancy. You could come back as lower-risk but lower-risk does not necessarily mean no risk [of having a child with Down's syndrome]. OK?

MRS LI: OK.

This extract highlights many points identified earlier in the book: the figuring of mothers-to-be as 'lower-risk or higher-risk', the significance of maternal age ('how old are you?'), the absence of Down's syndrome, the notion of non-directive care being difficult to uphold ('you might have to think whether having this test would be the best option'), and the naturalisation of screening practices. For my intentions here, I highlight Nicola's frequent allusions to termination. She cites termination on three occasions, using this to highlight the gravity of Mrs Li's decision-making and how delaying a diagnostic test will be increasingly problematic as the pregnancy progresses. However, the option of theoretically continuing a pregnancy following a diagnosis of Down's syndrome is never established. I observed similar occasions in other screening consultations, including those where parents-to-be with a higher-risk result of Down's syndrome were invited back to the clinic (Freymarsh specifically)[6] for counselling.

To refresh, if a diagnosis of Down's syndrome or another condition is suspected following screening at FAD or SAD, parents-to-be are offered diagnostic testing. If this is accepted, they are referred to FMD where this care is available free of charge (Dr Karman works in Springtown *and* FMD so is very likely to deal with such cases). After diagnostic testing, if a diagnosis of Down's syndrome is established, parents-to-be are offered a termination of pregnancy and are now under the care of FMD consultants. During one conversation, Dr Karman (FMD consultant) identifies some concerns after hypothetical prenatal diagnoses of Edward's syndrome or Patau syndrome:

> I think when there's a problem, some mothers feel abandoned and require support. Some midwives say 'well the foetus has Edward's [syndrome] or Patau [syndrome] and it's going to die so what can I do about it?' They forget there is still a woman here who is pregnant and has all of these concerns.

Dr Karman acknowledges how women feel abandoned in receipt of a diagnosis of Edward's syndrome (see: Thiele 2010) or Patau syndrome and, significantly for the claims made in this chapter, uses the term *foetus* when referring to these diagnoses. The following fieldnotes are taken from another conversation in which Dr Karman[7] uses similar language:

> Dr Karman, Roxanne (FMD sonographer), Robyn (FMD midwife) and Francine (FMD head midwife) are in the office. Dr Karman attended a hospital meeting yesterday where a range of obstetric professionals from Freymarsh and surrounding hospitals discussed 'the big issues in prenatal care'. Dr Karman recounts the event:

DR KARMAN: You wouldn't believe it. Maternity have more say in meetings over us. They had six main outcome factors: obesity, alcohol, breastfeeding, maternal satisfaction, caesarean, and good birth. So they talked about soft issues like breastfeeding, not stillbirth or foetal death. The focus has been completely lost. I was like 'Well the best thing is an alive mum and alive baby, and the next best thing is a well mum and well baby. And everything else comes after that.' You just can't believe it sometimes. They've lost the plot. They looked so horrified when I mentioned stillbirth and foetal death. There's too much emphasis on smoking, alcohol, breastfeeding, and all that. Everyone's concentrating on this and if they get the fluffy pink pram and that. They want all of the soft stuff, not the bad stuff. That part of the pregnancy is all fine but they have to think of the bad stuff too. The primary outcome should be a good healthy baby. You just don't know what will happen during screening and the extent of the many different problems until birth.

ROBYN: Exactly.

FRANCINE: Too right.

DR KARMAN: You can't win until afterwards. One percent of babies are born with CMV[8] where there are different severities. And it's not appropriate apparently. You can't tell them one in one-hundred babies will have CMV.

Dr Karman bemoans 'the focus' in pregnancy being exclusively on 'soft stuff', including breastfeeding and smoking, rather than the 'bad stuff', such as stillbirth and foetal death. Dr Karman's classification of 'bad stuff' reveals a distinction between 'foetal death' and 'a good healthy baby'. In an environment in which professionals 'can't win till [after childbirth]', Dr Karman opts for the term foetus over baby when discussing prospective death and/or termination.[9] This label is also embedded in clinical discourse once a potential condition is diagnosed and a termination of pregnancy is offered. That is, in FMD, once a termination of a pregnancy – for any condition – is considered to be a feasible option, discourses commonly shift from 'baby' to 'foetus'. Thus, it is here where the foetus/baby can be made and unmade. It is worth recognising here that the word 'foetus' itself is controversial:

> For obvious reasons, anti-abortionists prefer to use terms such as baby, or unborn child. In contrast, many feminists shy away from using the word baby, not wanting to give the foetus human status. There is a tendency to use the word foetus, although this leads to a further dilemma, as they recognise it to be a word that pregnant women themselves rarely use.
>
> (Williams 2002: 2085)

Many authors, particularly feminist scholars, have adopted a view of personhood as something which is constructed and negotiated as opposed to something which is inherent, suggesting that the biomedicalisation of pregnancy has supported the growing notion of foetal subjectivity (Howes-Mischel 2016). Departing from the dominance of a biomedical model of personhood, they recognise how parents, family and others can shift between the terms 'baby' and 'foetus' before, during, and after pregnancy (Condit 1995; Hopkins et al. 2005; Morgan 1996; Williams 2002), the latter concerning pregnancy loss (Layne 2003; Lotto 2015; Lovell 1997) and how 'the subject who is memorialised is a baby or child, rather than a foetus' (Keane 2009: 159); some foetuses are 'persons or "real babies", whereas others are not' (Layne 2003: 240). This is referred to by Morgan and Michaels (1999: 6) as 'person-making':

> Though the criteria governing the attribution of personhood are dynamic and subject to change, rituals and practices that govern person-making are extended to foetuses: foetuses are sexed, named, 'photographed', surgically altered, spoken to and about, and even speak themselves, Hollywood style.

This is particularly true of analyses around how ultrasound technology is a key site for the personification of the foetus or, rather, a human-in-waiting (Mitchell 2001); that is, how ultrasound transforms the foetus into a baby.[10] This shifting discourse and interpretation is exemplified in the words of Leah Rubinstein, a woman whose words act as an introduction to chapter 9 in Rapp's (2000: 220) seminal ethnography of prenatal testing in America:

> When we walked into the doctor's office, both my husband and I were crying. He looked up and said, 'What's wrong? Why are you both in tears?' 'It's our baby. Our baby is going to die,' I said. 'That isn't a baby,' he said firmly. 'It's a collection of cells that made a mistake.'

This shift between the different and interchangeable discourses of foetus and baby – thus demonstrating their 'legal, medical and social definitional difficulties' (Lovell 1997: 46) – has not been widely explored in relation to professionals' classificatory work and how they engage in such shifts. This is the focus for the remainder of this chapter with respect to how a possible termination of pregnancy is discussed in FMD. To repeat, in FMD, once a termination of a pregnancy – for any condition – is considered to be a feasible option, discourses frequently shift from using the term 'baby' to using the term 'foetus'. Thus, it is here where the baby/foetus can be made and unmade, and personhood can be ascribed or, possibly, revoked. The frailty and flexibility of the foetus/baby category is exemplified in a conversation between Victoria (SAD nurse) and Mrs John (mother-to-be) before an NT scan. When Victoria asks Mrs John 'so is this your first pregnancy?', she responds 'no but this is my first baby'. Mrs John indicates that in her prior pregnancy, ending in a miscarriage, there was no presence of a 'baby'. Instead, this current ('viable') foetus is afforded the status of baby. The following field-notes are taken from a discussion involving Dr Karman and Francine (FMD head midwife) of a possible 'feticide', an act that causes the death of a foetus prior to termination:

> DR KARMAN: [Walks into the office] This is not good. There's a feticide I have to organise for next week.
> FRANCINE: [Dejected] What a bad Friday.
> DR KARMAN: You're telling me. Placenta previa,[11] early pregnancy, feticide and induction of labour [medically induced abortion] but lots of bleeding if delivered. [...] She wants to terminate after twenty-four weeks and she's currently around twenty-three weeks in. The prognosis is very poor so we're going to recommend a feticide. This is not good.

Dr Karman, who is clearly upset, leaves the room. I ask Francine why the respective parents-to-be (Mr and Mrs Elton) want to terminate the pregnancy after twenty-four weeks:

FRANCINE: So the baby can be registered as a stillbirth rather than miscarriage which is easier for funerals. I think it makes the baby seem
more real.

Two minutes pass before Dr Karman returns to the silent office. Dr Karman
invites me to attend the feticide. The foetus has been diagnosed with a
'severe cardiac defect':

DR KARMAN: It's important for you Gareth because this screening and
termination is after twenty-one weeks and six days.[12] Sometimes this
happens with foetuses that have Down's syndrome. If they have a
cardiac scan, then a test, then terminating a foetus with Down's
[syndrome] can go beyond twenty-one weeks and six days. And to
terminate a foetus with Down's [syndrome] after twenty-one weeks
and six days is best through feticide.

I attend the procedure with Dr Karman. [...] Dr Karman refers to 'the
foetus' a few times during the procedure. Afterwards, I enter the office
with Dr Karman and Francine:

DR KARMAN: That was unusual. It's usually quicker and more straightforward than that. We usually inject potassium chloride into the left
ventricle inducing immediate asystole[13] and cardiac arrest but the
foetus was curled up.

Dr Karman and Francine reflect on a 'bad Friday' in FMD, with Francine
clarifying that Mr and Mrs Elton want a termination of pregnancy after
twenty-four weeks 'so the baby can be registered as a stillbirth rather than
miscarriage which is easier for funerals', an action that 'makes the baby seem
more real' (for further examples of this, see: Lotto 2015). Once more, the term
'foetus' is assumed throughout (the procedure itself is always referred to as a
'feticide', thus emphasising the word *foetus* over *baby*). For Lotto (2015) and
Olarte Sierra (2010), a foetus which is terminated can still 'become' a baby for
parents-to-be via memorials including ultrasound pictures, keeping ashes, and
organising funerals; 'choosing to interrupt a pregnancy does not necessarily
mean to re-interpret what was felt as a child into the term foetus' (Olarte
Sierra 2010: 206).[14] Whilst Olarte Sierra and Lotto claim that a termination
does not necessarily suggest such a shift (i.e. from the 'baby' to the 'foetus'),
the language used in FMD indicates that this *can* occur once a condition is
clinically defined as 'incompatible with life'.

How should we interpret this shift? Is it a purposeful move, or is it merely
an insignificant moment that does not merit critical attention? In the context
of this study, it seems to be the former. A possible reason for this shift, for
instance, is that it is a strategy used by professionals to hollow out the emo-
tionality of the term 'baby', both for parents-to-be and for themselves.

Consider the following conversation between Annie (FMD sonographer) and Francine (FMD head midwife) regarding the feticide case described above:

ANNIE: All the family are there [during the ultrasound scan that precedes the feticide] and [Mr Elton] was asking me to make out all these things as he couldn't. The eyes, head, heart, legs, and the Mum was like 'Ah, look at her all curled up.' They're such a lovely family, so supportive and close to one another. I don't often get affected by it but it's really hard sometimes.

FRANCINE: Yes, and it's not like you're heartless.

ANNIE: No definitely.

FRANCINE: You have to be detached.

ANNIE: Well you couldn't do this job if you didn't.

FRANCINE: Exactly. It's crazy because I'm crying at stuff on TV all the time but my son asks me if I cry when I give bad news. I mean not usually. I suppose it's just part of the job.

Annie and Francine outline the challenges of their work and how they must be 'detached'; without assuming emotional distance from both parents-to-be and the issues at hand, 'you couldn't do this job'. In an environment in which 'the unthinkable becomes a reality' (Chapter 3), professionals must adopt tactics to manage this emotional work. In their study of medical student training, Lief and Fox (1963) describe how the operating room's appearance and the serious conduct required of students justify and facilitate a technical and impersonal attitude to death. According to Lief and Fox (1963), body parts strongly connected with human qualities (face, genitalia, hands) are rarely dissected and tissues are depersonalised by removing a body from the room once an organ is removed. This allows students, Lief and Fox suggest, to approach their actions scientifically rather than emotionally, to develop a 'detached concern', which enables them to dissect a cadaver without disgust and listen empathetically to a patient without becoming emotionally involved. It is reasonable to suggest that in FMD, similarly, one method of maintaining moral and emotional distance from the issues at hand, to adopt a 'detached concern' (although professionals recognise that this is very difficult to do and that it is not possible to *completely* detach from their work), is figuratively shifting the baby to a foetus in certain moments.

'Disposing' of Down's syndrome

Once again, we may ask how Down's syndrome figures in this. In the previous extract describing the feticide, Dr Karman (FMD consultant) refers to a foetus, not baby, diagnosed with Down's syndrome. This technical discourse seems contrary to the positive accounts provided by professionals earlier in the book, namely Down's syndrome as being 'compatible with life' and as promising a 'good quality of life' (although I identified how such accounts were replaced during consultations with other discourses such as 'risk' and 'abnormality'). The following fieldnotes are taken from an interaction between Dr Karman and Robyn (FMD midwife) in the FMD office:

> Dr Karman enters the office following a consultation with Mr and Mrs Rose. I am handed a form by Dr Karman which contains details about Mr and Mrs Rose and the pregnancy:
>
> DR KARMAN: The foetus has a lateral ventriculomegaly.[15] [Mrs Rose] had a scan and it looks like two nerves are crossing over at the front of the brain. There is an agenesis of the corpus callosum[16] which means part of the brain is absent. It's a difficult consultation because it could be absolutely fine and the ventriculomegaly has no impact later on. But it could be associated with lissencephaly,[17] also known as smooth brain. That's associated with a real handicap and not handicapped like Down's [syndrome] where there is such a wide spectrum [of prognosis].
> ROBYN: Would you offer a termination with that?
> DR KARMAN: [Nods head] Yes. It's not really compatible with a good quality of life. It has associations with cerebral palsy[18] and other problems.

Dr Karman describes the case of a 'foetus' diagnosed with lateral ventriculomegaly and an agenesis of the corpus callosum, suggesting that this is a 'difficult consultation' owing to an uncertain prognosis. However, Dr Karman suspects the foetus could have lissencephaly, a condition 'associated with a real handicap' unlike Down's syndrome 'where there is such a wide spectrum [of prognosis]'. Finally, Dr Karman informs Robyn that a termination will be recommended since it is 'not really compatible with a good quality of life' and is indicative of 'other problems'.

Here, Dr Karman highlights how some conditions are not 'compatible with a good quality of life' and, in so doing, illuminates the role that medicine plays in categorising particular bodies/future bodies. Regardless of this categorical work, professionals cannot explicitly tell parents-to-be to terminate a pregnancy after a diagnosis of Down's syndrome specifically. There are two reasons for this. First, a strict adherence to the principles of informed choice and non-directive care emphasises that parents-to-be must make their own decisions independent of professional intervention. Notably, during one conversation, Dr Karman says that 'two out of three professionals will not perform a feticide beyond thirty-two weeks for Down's syndrome' since 'it is not seen as obstructing the quality of life' and 'it is ethically wrong to do a late amniocentesis if it's to determine whether to terminate or not'. This shows how professionals devise distinctions between whether a termination is appropriate or not with reference to the week of gestation. However, since most foetuses with Down's syndrome are diagnosed before thirty-two weeks gestation, the rhetoric of informed choice and non-directive care is drawn upon in such situations to reallocate responsibility for decision-making to parents-to-be.

Second, as Dr Karman claims, there is a 'wide spectrum' of the condition. This seems to be an irresolvable quandary for professionals and parents-to-be. Down's syndrome occupies a difficult position since it is enacted as 'compatible with life' yet can be offered as a legal reason for termination; how a baby will be fully affected by Down's syndrome is uncertain and, whilst the condition is likely to cause physical/mental limitations and a termination of pregnancy after a diagnosis is an option, the foetus is still described by professionals as viable. Elena (FMD head midwife) reflects upon this uncertainty during an interview:

> The question all parents ask before they make a decision about their pregnancy [and termination] is 'What sort of Down's baby will I have?' And this is another biggie which will help them make a decision. But there's no way of assessing abilities and a prognosis. But then you sort of say 'Well if you look at any child, you don't know their intelligence, their emotionality, you don't know.' I think it's that uncertainty which is the big push for some parents [to terminate], that unknown. I personally find that strange as all children are unknown. [...] And I'm sure there are a lot of parents, if this baby was sort of born out of the blue, they probably wouldn't [put him/her up for adoption] but it's because they have the choice [to terminate]. [...] I think people's perception of Down's syndrome is mostly from institutions still but I think what you put in is what you come out with, but that's true with any kid. But you've got to admire parents that go ahead with pregnancies after a Down's syndrome diagnosis, just as you admire parents who have to make that awful decision about not wanting to continue their pregnancies.

The inability to '[assess] abilities and a prognosis', according to Elena, is a 'big push' for some parents-to-be for terminating a pregnancy. Elena attempts to alleviate possible anxieties of parents-to-be by identifying how uncertainty surrounds any child's future, later suggesting that the negative image of Down's syndrome may still haunt reproductive practices but that she 'admires' those who either continue or terminate a pregnancy after a diagnosis. Elena's claim that the 'unknown' of Down's syndrome constitutes a reason why parents-to-be terminate the pregnancy also explains why the condition is inherently problematic for both parents-to-be and professionals. Its uncertainty, along with responsibility for choices being transferred to parents-to-be, ensures that Down's syndrome dwells in a betwixt and between state; the prognosis is uncertain, yet a termination is offered. This presents a thorny dilemma for professionals who must provide information to parents-to-be and concurrently negotiate the tricky terrain of deciding which situations constitute legal grounds for a termination.

One solution to settling this uncertainty is to categorise the entity diagnosed with Down's syndrome as a 'foetus'. Classification work is integral to preserving order in the clinic. Invisible yet imbricated in the everyday life of the prenatal clinic, such categorical work – difficult since 'people never easily fit into categories' (Bowker and Star 2000: 28) – powerfully orders interactions and becomes crucial for marking out what is 'normal' and 'abnormal'. In the case of Down's syndrome, professionals' accounts suggest the condition is characte-ristic of what Douglas (1966: 38) refers to as an 'ambiguity' or 'anomaly' (not in the sense of being a genetic 'anomaly' as clinically defined); an ambiguity is 'a character of statements capable of two interpretations', whilst an anomaly is 'an element which does not fit a given set or series'. Douglas says there is little advantage on making distinctions between these two terms in their practical application (as such, I will be using the terms interchangeably). She adds that, as social life rarely conforms to simple categories, any given classifica-tion system must give rise to anomalies and 'any given culture must confront events which seem to defy its assumptions' (1966: 40). Thus, we must reflect with profit on our main classifications and how we treat those things that cannot fit them (Douglas outlines several methods of treating an anomaly). One example used by Douglas is cited from Evans-Pritchard's (1956) work on how the Nuer[19] treat babies with anatomical defects as baby hippopotamuses accidently born to humans.[20] Since they obscure the distinction between human and non-human, placing them in the river dismisses the indefinable and 'affirms and strengthens the definitions to which they do not conform' (Douglas 1966: 40).

Similar gestures of separation and classification emerge in FMD. Profes-sionals frequently 'confront' the anomaly of Down's syndrome – as a condition that is compatible with life and which professionals (in the clinic's backstage) often describe positively, yet is also grounds for legally terminating a pregnancy – by settling on a universal interpretation of it as an abnormality. Since it is 'likely to confuse or contradict cherished classifications', the condition is 'fitted' into the rigid category of abnormality so that it does not disturb, and confirms confidence in, classifications already established in the prenatal clinic – namely, between normal and abnormal (Douglas 1966: 37–38). By referring to the 'foetus' with Down's syndrome, and by categorising the condition itself as an abnormality in the frontstage of the clinic (i.e. without full reference to its variability and uncertain prognosis, thus reducing its ambiguity), profes-sionals can enact the 'disposal' (Berg 1992; Hillman 2007; Latimer 1997; Munro 2001) of Down's syndrome to 'reorganise the environment' (Douglas 1966: 2). In prenatal medicine, the 'search for anomalies [...] may undermine claims to foetal personhood' (Roberts 2012: 301). What I argue is that in

FMD, a diagnosis of Down's syndrome – an ambiguous entity, as outlined above – ensures that what was possibly classified previously as a baby (e.g. via ultrasound) is likely to be classified as a 'foetus', and that what is recognised by professionals as a complex and variable condition is, instead, confined within the stiff and narrowing classification of abnormality. Together with providing parents-to-be and professionals with a mechanism to try to accomplish moral/emotional distance from the term *baby*, this move also allows for the disposal of Down's syndrome. This reaffirms categories as natural and valid (and fixed), restores order, and settles ambiguities in the prenatal clinic – and, in turn, makes a termination of pregnancy possible.

The cleft board

This analysis of how the foetus/baby status can be made and unmade extends to the materiality of FMD and specifically the 'cleft board', a large picture-board that is adorned on a wall in the FMD waiting room. Professionals ask parents-to-be, post-childbirth, to return to the department and supply photographs of their baby diagnosed with a cleft lip/palate and/or congenital condition (e.g. spina bifida) to display on this board. The following fieldnotes are taken from a consultation between Dr Karman (FMD consultant), Elena (FMD midwife), and Mr and Mrs Hunt (parents-to-be) with respect to a diagnosis of an abnormal aortic arch in the foetus[21]:

DR KARMAN: So would you like a late amniocentesis?

MRS HUNT: I plan not to because I want to concentrate on the heart side of things. And I've heard from a few of the people that if something was wrong, a number of other problems would have been detected by now.

DR KARMAN: Not in all cases do all other problems show up in the scans or diagnostic tests. The heart is linked to other stuff but this may be the only sign. A heart defect will indicate abnormality in 5% of cases and the only way you can know whether there are any problems is by an amniocentesis. But the likelihood is that the baby's chromosomal development is normal. That's 95% likely [Dr Karman smiles. Mr and Mrs Hunt smile back].

ELENA: You should book an appointment to come here again so we can keep an eye on everything.

DR KARMAN: Yes [Mr and Mrs Hunt nod]. Can you bring baby into the department after he or she is born?

MRS HUNT: Sure.

MR HUNT: Of course.

DR KARMAN: I'd like to add a photograph of him or her to the [cleft] board.

ELENA: Yes. If something is wrong, it's good for parents to see a picture with the problem and see that there is still a baby here.

DR KARMAN: Absolutely [smiles at Mr and Mrs Hunt].

MRS HUNT: Yes it's nice to know that you're [slightly pauses].
DR KARMAN: [Interrupting] It's nice to see the baby ahead of the problem.
ELENA: Definitely.
MRS HUNT: Definitely. It's nice to see that you're not on your own.

Dr Karman's response to Mrs Hunt's rejection of amniocentesis is arguably directive, potentially inciting anxiety in Mr and Mrs Hunt by claiming that 'other problems' may be hidden and the diagnostic test would establish an absence or presence of 'abnormality' (though Dr Karman attempts to repair this by recognising that a 'normal' baby development is '95% likely'). Dr Karman also asks Mr and Mrs Hunt if they would bring their newborn baby into FMD so that a photograph can be taken and added to the cleft board. If 'something is wrong', Elena deduces, other parents-to-be in a similar situation will benefit from seeing 'that there is still a baby here'. Dr Karman says that 'it's nice to see the baby ahead of the problem' before Mrs Hunt adds 'it's nice to see that you're not on your own'. During an interview, Francine (FMD head midwife) highlights the importance of the cleft board:

> I think [the cleft board] is for women to come in and see their babies could be diagnosed with certain abnormalities but at the end of the day, they still look normal. I think because you can't see your baby apart from through the black and white images [via ultrasound scan], a lot of women picture some horrific things in their mind. Babies have gastroschisis[22] or spina bifida and they have images of these huge messes when in fact you're looking at something really small. So I think it's just to get things into perspective. So if we say 'baby's got a cleft' or whatever, and they say 'what's that going to look like', you can show them a picture and say 'this looks like a normal baby'. At the end of the day, it might have a structural problem but it will look like a normal baby. The other toss of the coin is that women terminate because of abnormalities and they say to me 'what will my baby look like?' when they deliver having terminated the pregnancy and I say, 'well, it will look normal'. If they terminated a pregnancy for a brain abnormality, the baby will look normal and I think that's quite hard because a woman will have at the back of her mind 'did I do the right thing? I know they're telling me it did have brain abnormalities but did it, and would it really be affected that way?' And it could be the same with Down's syndrome. They might terminate and look at the baby when the baby's born and think 'he doesn't look very Down's syndrome, have they got it right, was it just a mildly affected Down's [syndrome baby], and could we have coped with it?'

Francine's account begins by her identifying the cleft board as beneficial for mothers-to-be to see that 'their babies could be diagnosed with certain abnormalities but at the end of the day, they still look normal'. Since many parents-to-be 'picture some horrific things' if receiving a diagnosis, the cleft board represents a normalising technology that helps 'get things into perspective' by revealing a baby which 'will look like a normal baby'. Similar normalising technologies include offering 4D baby bonding scans free-of-charge to parents-to-be after a diagnosis of cleft lip/palate or another structural defect (these are offered at SAD/FMD but only take place at SAD – see: Thomas 2015). The cleft board, together with the 4D scans, reveal the importance of (visual) 'normality' to parents-to-be, with normality being constituted as a perceived visual absence of *ab*normality. Interestingly, there is no picture of a newborn baby with Down's syndrome adorning the cleft board. In an interview, Elena (FMD head midwife) reflects on this, together with the board's value:

> Parents look at it all the time and the most positive thing we've ever done here is put that up. But the only thing we haven't got up there is Down's [syndrome] because parents don't send pictures back of their Down's babies.

Elena perceives the cleft board as allowing parents-to-be to frame their baby in a positive light by, as she articulates during the consultation with Mr and Mrs Hunt (cited earlier in this chapter), 'see[ing] there is a still a baby there'. For workers at Freymarsh, the board – aligned with talk – not only encourages public displays of the satisfaction of parents-to-be with the service but can also help 'normalise' a foetus/baby by playing to a child's future normality (Silverman 1987). I have already identified how the Down's syndrome 'face' (Latimer 2013), corresponding to the distinctive facial features caused by the condition, can signify a failure to fulfil expectations in the pursuit of perfection in a pregnancy outcome. Elena's and Francine's accounts, taken together, suggest that a picture of a newborn baby with Down's syndrome may transform perceptions of parents-to-be and re-normalise the baby (at least an artificial/ aesthetic normality). Yet the absence of Down's syndrome on the board, ironically, reflects its absence in screening consultations.

I argue that the absence of a Down's syndrome presence on the board relates to the denigrating portrayal of the condition which is accomplished in everyday clinical life. In the early stages of prenatal care, Down's syndrome is subjected to narrow and universalising constitutions of 'risk' and 'abnorm-ality' whilst, in FMD, the term 'foetus' is often used when discussing a possible termination of pregnancy for the condition. Returning to the case of Mr and Mrs Hunt, the 'viability' of their foetus/baby allows Dr Karman to make a move to re-normalise their baby after the diagnosis. Since a chromo-somal abnormality is unlikely, and so a termination will not be offered, the status of 'baby' is retained and an invitation to submit a photograph to be placed onto the cleft board is tendered. In contrast, when the foetus/baby has or is suspected of having Down's syndrome, the baby is often transformed into a foetus. Such moves restore the local order, namely by settling the ambiguous category of Down's syndrome (as 'viable' but as something one screens, tests, and possibly terminates for) and reinforcing the boundary between normal (babies) and abnormal (foetuses). This, in turn, allows for the effective disposal of a foetus with the condition in prenatal care.

Summary

In this chapter, I explored how Down's syndrome screening can promote a notion of perfectibility that shapes understandings of disability. The pursuit of perfection in reproductive outcomes is largely framed through the lens of the visual, with Down's syndrome – with respect to its 'face' – being constituted as a negative outcome. This also implicates mothers-to-be and particularly those at an 'advanced maternal age' who, throughout pregnancy, are embroiled in cultural ideologies of perfection/normality that may cause them to undertake screening (i.e. to *promise* 'normality') and that may cause feelings of blame and responsibility if there is any deviation in the expected outcome. Finally, it was shown how this notion of normality emerges in the categorical work of professionals in FMD. The foetus with Down's syndrome occupies a between-and-betwixt state as it is recognised as 'compatible with life' yet the condition can be used as a reason for terminating a pregnancy. In order to rectify this situation, FMD professionals – once a diagnosis is provided or suspected – can transform the (normal) 'baby' into the (abnormal) 'foetus'. This discursive work, by reducing the ambiguity of Down's syndrome (as acknowledged by the professionals), restores order and reaffirms the boundary between normal and abnormal in the clinic. Just as Foucault (1983) presses that there is no madness without reason, there is no abnormal without normal in prenatal care. A combination of all of these factors – the value placed on producing perfection during pregnancy, an imperative for mothers-to-be to eliminate all 'risks', and the making and unmaking of the foetus/baby – all contribute to the routinisation of Down's syndrome screening and the configuring of the condition, in frontstage consultations, as a negative outcome. In the concluding chapter, I identify how focusing on one specific aspect of medical work (prenatal screening) raises many important questions for medicine and wider society.

Notes

1 Anencephaly is a cephalic condition resulting from a neural tube defect in which a major portion of the brain, skull, or scalp is absent. With few exceptions, most babies with anencephaly will not survive birth.
2 Spina bifida is a congenital developmental condition caused by the incomplete closing of a neural tube.
3 As a reminder, the pictures show a young father smiling and holding his newborn child. Both are photographed underwater. Lisa (SAD sonographer) explains that newborn babies have a natural diving reflex and so avoid inhaling water into their lungs.

4 The idea of bonding is central to maternal discourses. In the age of prenatal technologies, maternal attachment – once considered 'natural' – seemingly cannot be left to nature and women (Mitchell and Georges 1997).

5 I realise that this analysis is based on hetero-normative assumptions about partnerships. Only one consultation I observed involved a same-sex couple (Springtown). In this case, it would be more correct to say screening implicates the 'carrier' of the baby.

6 In Springtown, parents-to-be receive higher-risk results via telephone. This is primarily done by Francine who also works at FMD. She often telephones these parents-to-be at night from her home, and so observing these telephone calls was unfeasible.

7 Many of the extracts cite Dr Karman since there are only two practising consultants in FMD. Dr Karman, as one of these consultants, deals with the vast majority of cases that I observed.

8 CMV (cytomegalovirus) is a virus which can be transmitted to a foetus before birth. It is a common cause of birth defects and has a range of severities.

9 In England and Wales, under the Abortion Act (1967), abortions can only be carried out in a hospital or specialist licensed clinic. The NHS (2014) states that the method of abortion depends on the length of a pregnancy. Methods include early medical abortion (up to nine weeks of pregnancy), vacuum aspiration or suction termination (from seven to fifteen weeks of pregnancy), late medical abortion (from nine to twenty weeks of pregnancy), surgical dilation and evacuation (from fifteen weeks of pregnancy), and late abortion (from twenty to twenty-four weeks of pregnancy). There are two options for late abortion: surgical two-stage abortion and medically induced abortion.

10 Although many authors have described how ultrasound imagery contributes to personifying the foetus (Krøløkke 2011; Mitchell 2001), others identify more ambivalent experiences of pregnancy loss, abortion, and maternal–foetal bonding via ultrasound (Beynon-Jones 2015; Kimport 2012).

11 Placenta previa is a complication in which the placenta is inserted partially or wholly in the lower uterine segment. It is the largest cause of antepartum haemorrhage (vaginal bleeding).

12 In FMD, the recommended gestation after which feticide should be offered as part of a termination of pregnancy is twenty-one weeks and six days gestation (Springtown do not offer this service as they are not equipped to perform this procedure).

13 Asystole is a state of no cardiac electrical activity (colloquially known as flatline) which may be one of the conditions used to certify clinical or legal death.

14 Lotto (2015) says that whilst humanising a 'foetus' to take on the identity of a 'baby' can offer comfort and a rite of passage to social rituals of grief (e.g. funerals), the public recognition of a termination can also cause feelings of stigma and shame.

15 Ventriculomegaly is a brain condition which occurs when the lateral ventricles become dilated. It occurs in around 1% of pregnancies.

16 Agenesis of the corpus callosum is a rare birth defect in which there is a partial or complete absence of the corpus callosum, the band of white matter connecting the two hemispheres in the brain.

17 Lissencephaly is a rare brain defect caused by defective neuronal migration during the twelfth and twenty-fourth week of gestation. It is a form of cephalic disorder, meaning congenital conditions stemming from damage to, or abnormal development of, the budding nervous system.

18 Cerebral palsy is a blanket term covering a range of neurological conditions which affect a child's movement and coordination.

19 The Nuer are a Nilotic ethnic group primarily inhabiting the Nile Valley in southern Sudan.
20 This is just one example of how people have attempted to influence, or rectify, reproductive outcomes throughout human history via religious rituals and medical interventions that aim to assure a healthy baby and/or birth (for further examples, see: Gammeltoft and Wahlberg 2014).
21 The aortic arch is the portion of the main artery in the human heart between the ascending and descending aorta.
22 Gastroschisis is a congenital defect characterised by a structural defect in the abdominal wall through which the abdominal contents protrude.

Bibliography

Alderson, P. 2001. Down's syndrome: cost, quality and value of life. *Social Science and Medicine* 53(5), pp. 627–638.

Beynon-Jones, S. 2015. Re-visioning ultrasound through women's account of pre-abortion care in England. *Gender and Society* 29(5), pp. 694–715.

Berg, M. 1992. The construction of medical disposals: medical sociology and medical problem solving in clinical practice. *Sociology of Health and Illness* 14(2), pp. 151–180.

Bowker, G.C. and Star, S.L. 2000. *Sorting Things Out: Classification and Its Consequences*. Cambridge, MA: MIT Press.

Buchbinder, M. and Timmermans, S. 2012. Medical technologies and the dream of the perfect newborn. *Medical Anthropology* 30(1), pp. 56–80.

Budds, K., Locke, A. and Burr, V. 2013. 'Risky business': constructing the 'choice' to 'delay' motherhood in the British press. *Feminist Media Studies* 13(1), pp. 132–147.

Canguilhem, G. 2005. Monstrosity and the monstrous. In: Fraser, M. and Greco, M. eds. *The Body: A Reader*. London: Routledge, pp. 187–193.

Condit, D. 1995. Foetal personhood: political identity under construction. In: Boiling, P. ed. *Expecting Trouble: Surrogacy, Foetal Abuse and New Reproductive Technologies*. Boulder, CO: Westview Press, pp. 25–54.

Dimond, R. 2013. Negotiating identity at the intersection of paediatric and genetic medicine: the parent as facilitator, narrator and patient. *Sociology of Health and Illness* 36(1), pp. 1–14.

Douglas, M. 1966. *Purity and Danger: An Analysis of the Concepts of Pollution and Taboo*. London: Routledge and Kegan Paul.

Douglas, M. 1992. *Risk and Blame: Essays in Cultural Theory*. London: Routledge.

Evans-Pritchard, E.E. 1956. *Nuer Religion*. Oxford: Oxford University Press.

Foucault, M. 1979. *Discipline and Punish: The Birth of the Prison*. Harmondsworth: Penguin.

Foucault, M. 1983. The subject and power. In: Dreyfus, H.L. and Rabinow, P. eds. *Michel Foucault: Beyond Structuralism and Hermeneutics*. Chicago: University of Chicago Press, pp. 208–226.

Gammeltoft, T.M. 2007. Prenatal diagnosis in postwar Vietnam: power, subjectivity, and citizenship. *American Anthropologist* 109(1), pp. 153–163.

Gammeltoft, T. and Wahlberg, A. 2014. Selective reproductive technologies. *Annual Review of Anthropology* 43, pp. 201–216.

García, E., Timmermans, D.R.M. and van Leeuwen, E. 2012. Parental duties and prenatal screening: does an offer of prenatal screening lead women to believe that they are morally compelled to test? *Midwifery* 28(6), pp. 837–843.

Goffman, E. 1963. *Stigma: Notes on the Management of Spoiled Identity*. New York: Simon and Schuster.

Gottfreðsdóttir, H., Björnsdóttir, K. and Sandall, J. 2009. 'This is just what you do when you are pregnant': a qualitative study of prospective parents in Iceland who accept nuchal translucency screening. *Midwifery* 25(6), pp. 711–720.

Greco, M. 1993. Psychosomatic subjects and the 'duty to be well': personal agency within medical rationality. *Economy and Society* 22(3), pp. 357–372.

Gross, S.E. 2010. 'The alien baby': risk, blame and prenatal indeterminacy. *Health, Risk and Society* 12(1), pp. 21–31.

Hill, A. and Asthana, A. 2009. Women urged to test for fertility at 30 [Online]. Available at: www.theguardian.com/lifeandstyle/2009/aug/09/fertility-mot-children-nhs [Accessed: 7 August 2016].

Hillman, A. 2007. *Negotiating Access: Practices of Inclusion and Exclusion in the Performance of 'Real' Emergency Medicine*. Unpublished Ph.D. Thesis, Cardiff University.

HM Government. 2016. Abortion Act 1967 [Online]. Available at: www.legislation.gov.uk/ukpga/1967/87/section/1 [Accessed: 7 August 2016].

Hopkins, N., Zeedyk, S. and Raitt, F. 2005. Visualising abortion: emotion discourse and foetal imagery in a contemporary abortion debate. *Social Science and Medicine* 61(2), pp. 393–403.

Horlick-Jones, T. 2005. On 'risk work': professional discourse, accountability, and everyday action. *Health, Risk and Society* 7(3), pp. 293–307.

Howes-Mischel, R. 2016. 'With this you can meet your baby': foetal personhood and audible heartbeats in Oaxacan public health. *Medical Anthropology Quarterly* 30(2), pp. 186–202.

Ivry, T. 2006. At the backstage of prenatal care: Japanese ob-gyns negotiating prenatal diagnosis. *Medical Anthropology Quarterly* 20(4), pp. 441–468.

Keane, H. 2009. Foetal personhood and representations of the absent child in pregnancy loss memorialization. *Feminist Theory* 10(2), pp. 153–171.

Kimport, K. 2012. (Mis)understanding abortion regret. *Symbolic Interaction* 35(2), pp. 105–122.

Kr¸løkke, C. 2011. Biotourist performances: doing parenting during the ultrasound. *Text and Performance Quarterly* 31(1), pp. 15–36.

Landsman, G. 1998. Reconstructing motherhood in the age of 'perfect' babies: mothers of infants and toddlers with disabilities. *Signs* 24(1), pp. 69–99.

Landsman, G. 2009. *Reconstructing Motherhood and Disability in the Age of 'Perfect' Babies: Lives of Mothers of Infants and Toddlers with Disabilities*. New York: Routledge.

Latimer, J.E. 1997. Giving patients a future: the constituting of classes in an acute medical unit. *Sociology of Health and Illness* 19(2), pp. 160–185.

Latimer, J.E. 2007. Diagnosis, dysmorphology, and the family: knowledge, motility, choice. *Medical Anthropology* 26(2), pp. 97–138.

Latimer, J.E. 2013. *The Gene, the Clinic and the Family: Diagnosing Dysmorphology, Reviving Medical Dominance*. London: Routledge.

Layne, L. 2003. *Motherhood Lost: A Feminist Account of Pregnancy and Loss in America*. London: Routledge.

Lief, H.I. and Fox, R.C. 1963. The medical student's training for detached concern. In: Lief, H.I., Lief, V.F. and Lief, N.R. eds. *The Psychological Basis of Medical Practice*. New York: Harper and Row, pp. 12–35.

Lotto, R. 2015. *Decision Making About Congenital Anomalies: How do Women and Their Partners Make the Decision to Continue or Terminate a Pregnancy Following Suspicion or Diagnosis of a Severe Congenital Anomaly?* Unpublished Ph.D. Thesis, University of Leicester.

Lovell, A. 1997. Death at the beginning of life. In: Field, D., Hockey, J. and Small, N. eds. *Death, Gender and Ethnicity*. London: Routledge, pp. 29–51.

Lupton, D. 2013. *The Social Worlds of the Unborn*. Basingstoke: Palgrave Macmillan.

McLaughlin, J. 2003. Screening networks: shared agendas in feminist and disability movement challenges to antenatal screening and abortion. *Disability and Society* 18 (3), pp. 297–310.

Mitchell, L.M. 2001. *Baby's First Picture: Ultrasound and the Politics of Fetal Subjects*. Toronto: University of Toronto Press.

Mitchell, L.M. and Georges, E. 1997. Cross-cultural cyborgs: Greek and Canadian women's discourses on fetal ultrasound. *Feminist Studies* 23(2), pp. 373–401.

Morgan, L.M. 1996. Foetal relationality in feminist philosophy: an anthropological critique. *Hypatia* 11(3), pp. 47–70.

Morgan, L.M. and Michaels, M.W. 1999. *Foetal Subjects, Feminist Positions*. Philadelphia: University of Pennsylvania Press.

Müller-Rockstroh, B. 2011. Foetuses, facts and frictions: insights from ultrasound research in Tanzania. In: Geissler, P.W. and Molyneux, C. eds. *Evidence, Ethos and Experiment: The Anthropology and History of Medical Research in Africa*. New York: Berghahn Books, pp. 245–262.

Munro, R. 2001. Disposal of the body: upending postmodernism. *Ephemera* 1(2), pp. 108–130.

NHS. 2014. Abortion: how is it performed. *NHS Choices* [Online]. Available at: www.nhs.uk/Conditions/Abortion/Pages/How-is-it-performed.aspx [Accessed: 7 August 2016].

Olarte Sierra, M.F. 2010. *Achieving the Desirable Nation: Abortion and Antenatal Testing in Colombia (the Case of Amniocentesis)*. Unpublished Ph.D. Thesis, University of Amsterdam.

Possamai-Inesedy, A. 2006. Confining risk: choice and responsibility in childbirth within a risk society. *Health Sociology Review* 15(4), pp. 406–414.

Rapp, R. 1995. Hereditary, or revising the facts of life. In: Delaney, C. and Yanagisako, S. eds. *Naturalizing Power: Essays in Feminist Cultural Analysis*. London: Routledge, pp. 69–86.

Rapp, R. 1999. Foreword. In: Layne, L.L. ed. *Transformative Motherhood: On Giving and Getting in a Consumer Culture*. New York: New York University Press, pp. xi–xix.

Rapp, R. 2000. *Testing Women, Testing the Fetus: The Social Impact of Amniocentesis in America*. London: Routledge.

Reed, K. 2012. *Gender and Genetics: Sociology of the Prenatal*. London: Routledge.

Remennick, L. 2006. The quest for the perfect baby: why do Israeli women seek prenatal genetic testing? *Sociology of Health and Illness* 28(1), pp. 21–53.

Roberts, J. 2012. 'Wakey wakey baby': narrating four-dimensional (4D) bonding scans. *Sociology of Health and Illness* 34(2), pp. 299–314.

Rothman, B.K. 1986. *The Tentative Pregnancy: Amniocentesis and the Sexual Politics of Motherhood*. London: Pandora.

Rothman, B.K. 1998. *Genetic Maps and Human Imaginations: The Limits of Science in Understanding Who We Are*. New York: Norton.

Shakespeare, T.W. 2000. Arguing about genetics and disability. *Interaction* 13(3), pp. 11–14.

Silverman, D. 1987. *Communication and Medical Practice: Social Relations in the Clinic.* London: Sage.

Taylor, J.S. 2008. *The Public Life of the Fetal Sonogram: Technology, Consumption and the Politics of Reproduction.* New Brunswick, NJ: Rutgers University Press.

Thiele, P. 2010. He was my son, not a dying baby. *Journal of Medical Ethics* 36(11), pp. 646–647.

Thomas, G.M. 2014. Cooling the mother out: revisiting and revising Goffman's account. *Symbolic Interaction* 37(2), pp. 283–299.

Thomas, G.M. 2015. Picture perfect: '4D' ultrasound and the commoditisation of the private prenatal clinic. *Journal of Consumer Culture* [Online first].

Thomas, G.M. and Lupton, D. 2016. Threats and thrills: pregnancy apps, risk, and consumption. *Health, Risk and Society* 17(7–8), pp. 495–509.

Timmermans, S. and Buchbinder, M. 2010. Patients-in-waiting: living between sickness and health in the genomics era. *Journal of Health and Social Behaviour* 51(4), pp. 408–423.

Timmermans, S. and Shostak, S. 2016. Gene worlds. *Health* 20(1), pp. 33–48.

Williams, C. 2002. Framing the foetus in medical work: rituals and practices. *Social Science and Medicine* 60(9), pp. 2085–2095.

Wolf, J.B. 2011. *Is Breast Best?: Taking on the Breastfeeding Experts and the New High Stakes of Motherhood.* New York: New York University Press.

Chapter 7

Keeping the back door ajar?

In the preceding chapters, I explored how a particular biomedical practice – screening for Down's syndrome – is routinised as a 'normal' component of prenatal care and how the condition itself is negatively constituted in the mundane, everyday practices of the clinic. Drawing heavily upon observations of frontstage screening consultations, I began my analysis in Chapter 3 by exploring how screening is organised and how it is downgraded by professionals as a trivial, non-prioritised task in three interrelated ways. First, the task of doing screening, at least initially, is relegated from consultants to midwives and sonographers, allowing the former to defend disciplinary boundaries and protect the purity of the clinic. Consultants only attach to Down's syndrome screening once a diagnosis and potential termination is possible whilst midwives and sonographers, contrastingly, appear reluctantly attached. Second, professionals define screening, both inside and outside of consultations, as a routine affair. This is accomplished through social practices, such as describing screening as 'simple' and 'just a chat', and through the materiality and space of the clinic, such as the use of doors and rooms. Third, professionals classify Down's syndrome screening consultations as a dull, repetitive, and valueless task that does not permit the performance of an authentic professional role. Whilst responsible for delivering this programme, they minimise the value of screening by privileging other tasks, namely 'hands-on work', that aligns with work-based expectations. This downgrading work, in turn, leads to screening being routinely embedded and stabilised as a 'normal' moment in prenatal care.

This analysis was extended in Chapter 4 to identify two more ways in which Down's syndrome screening is sedimented as a routine part of prenatal care. First, whilst professionals convey private misgivings about screening in the backstage of the clinic, the entangling rhetoric of 'informed choice' and 'non-directive care' constitutes a resource that allows professionals to detach from, and 'dispose' of, screening. In the frontstage of prenatal care, professionals allocate full responsibility for decision-making to parents-to-be. This shifts accountability (and, subsequently, blame) and accomplishes screening again as a 'normal' part of pregnancy. Second, screening is routinised by the 'social' dimensions of ultrasound scans (and particularly NT scans) being privileged over its 'medical' dimensions. Ultrasound scans, in such moments, are reconstructed as a 'day out' to welcome a new family member. This often trumps the medical agenda – that of prenatally detecting potential concerns with a foetus or pregnant woman. Whilst the medical dimensions of the NT scan are discussed, its social dimensions are widely promoted and its value as a serious procedure is, therefore, simultaneously diminished. Such situations produce circumstances in which screening is downgraded and, in turn, naturalised as a routine pregnancy practice. In addition, producing a 'baby' (not a 'foetus') for parents-to-be to gaze at – a baby with distinctive behaviours and physical features affiliated with personality traits and gendered conduct – contributes to the configuring of certain types of 'normal' bodies (Vailly 2008).

I built on this idea in Chapter 5 by exploring how Down's syndrome itself is constituted inside and outside of screening encounters. Professionals often express another concern with screening by describing Down's syndrome as 'compatible with life', a catch-all term signifying that someone with the condition can survive birth and enjoy a good 'quality of life'. However, whilst in the clinic's 'backstage' professionals describe the condition in positive terms and use this to express their own ambiguities about screening, such values and interpretations – and a wider discussion of Down's syndrome – are made absent in consultations. I explained that this corresponds to the familiarity of Down's syndrome to the UK public, the organisation of care, and a lack of knowledge about the condition among several professionals. Instead, the condition becomes present both inside and outside consultations via a dominant yet implicit discourse which associates the condition with 'risk' and its ancillary categories of 'problem', 'bad news', and 'abnormality'. Professionals do not overtly identify the 'miserable lives of people with disabilities', like the geneticists in Kerr et al.'s (1998: 181) research, yet they, instead, subtly and (I believe) unintentionally construct Down's syndrome as a negative pregnancy outcome. Rather than acknowledging the variability and complexity of the condition, as sometimes expressed in the clinic's backstage, professionals confine the condition to a narrowing, universalising, and purely technical definition of being outside the 'normal' (an example is the offer of screening for Down's syndrome alongside a range of 'diseases').

Chapter 6, the final chapter to present empirical data, extended this analysis by identifying how negative constitutions of Down's syndrome pertain to cultural ideologies around 'ab/normality' and 'im/perfection' that emerge in the social and material life of the clinic. This institutes mothers-to-be, particularly those of an 'advanced maternal age', as primarily responsible for accomplishing flawlessness in a foetus/baby that may lead them, in effect, to interpret screening as an instance of conformity and a chance to eliminate any 'risks' flagged up in prenatal care. Here, the responsible mother is she 'who does everything – takes all tests – to ensure foetal health' (Lippman 1994: 22). Finally, the chapter examined how Down's syndrome and ideals of 'normality' are enacted by discursive shifts between 'foetus' and 'baby' after a Down's syndrome diagnosis, as both category and process, is established or largely suspected. Down's syndrome is a contestable condition in the 'grey area' since it has an uncertain prognosis (as described by consultants, among others) but can be used as a reason for a termination of pregnancy. As such, there are contradictions and uncertainties that require resolution in the clinic. This ambiguity is resolved, in turn, by settling on the term 'foetus' which denies a 'baby' its personhood, thereby making a termination of pregnancy possible. This allows professionals and parents-to-be to both accomplish emotional and moral distance from the foetus/baby and restore order in the clinic by reinforcing the boundaries between normal (babies) and abnormal (foetuses). To conclude, it was suggested that by bringing ideals of what is normal/perfect close to hand, these elements position both parents-to-be and the born/unborn child with Down's syndrome in certain ways.

In sum, my book contributes to accounts around how medical work is organised and performed in everyday routines (Bosk 1992; Latimer 2000; Silverman 1987; Strong 1979) and how values around disability intersect with reproductive technologies (Ettorre 2002; Ginsburg and Rapp 1995; 2013; Ivry 2006; Landsman 1998; 2009; Latimer 2013; Lippman 1994; Parens and Asch 2000; Rapp 2000; Rothman 1986; Rothschild 2005; Shakespeare 1999; Vailly 2008; 2014; Vassy et al. 2014; Wasserman and Asch 2006). It also extends the field in three explicit ways. First, it draws on ethnographic data that is frequently missing in research on Down's syndrome screening, simultaneously identifying the shifts between professionals' accounts and what happens in everyday clinical practice. My ethnography of two healthcare institutions, thus, champions using observational fieldwork in explicating the implicit and exposing the taken-for-granted affairs of everyday life. Second, it supports the call to expose and unpack the neat and narrow category of 'disability' that discounts the many complexities and contradictions of different conditions, such as Down's syndrome, and that avoids a thorough dissection of how these categories/diagnoses are negotiated in the everyday practices of the clinic. Third, I identify the value of theoretical pluralism – implicitly if not always explicitly – for analysing the mundane and ordinary routines deeply embedded in the fabric of medical work that produce and reproduce certain power relations and cultural values. Informed by theoretical work which provides sturdy foundations for attending to the complex interplay of practices, discourses, and materials, the book deconstructs one of the most routine and taken-for-granted aspects of pregnancy in the UK.

Generally, my book shows how medicine is accomplished in ritual and mundane forms. Less generally, I highlight how Down's syndrome screening represents a routine practice which has transformed obstetric medicine, invigorated parental expectations, shaped issues surrounding the politics of reproduction, and reproduced certain body–society relations. I have drawn explicit attention to social practices and cultural materials in which alignments are made, accounts are produced, categorisations are erected and mutated, identities are accomplished, and knowledge is produced in local settings. This allows for the production of soft data which, as shown, raises hard questions about some of the most profound dilemmas of our time. In so doing, I show how Down's syndrome occupies a rather odd position in the clinic. There are inherent shifts – I borrow and employ the term 'motility' when referring to this throughout the book – in the (backstage) accounts of professionals and (frontstage) screening consultations. These shifts are certainly not interpreted as contradictions, deviancies, or unguarded statements which involve professionals 'slipping up' and cancelling out other pronouncements. Rather, they are interpreted as examples of how professionals shift backward and forward between distinct discursive forms – and for different reasons. Early in Down's syndrome screening, for instance, consultants do not attach themselves to the practice as it has yet to reach the status of clinical interest. In order to protect the purity of the clinic, this particular duty is relegated to midwives and sonographers who, interestingly, similarly detach themselves from screening since it does not constitute 'hands-on work'. Arguably, then, screening in Freymarsh and Springtown becomes 'matter out of place' (Douglas 1966).

What is more, this motility emerges in how midwives (at least, more than sonographers) claim that they do not 'do pathology' yet spend most of their time monitoring and probing mothers-to-be in a cycle of clinically oriented surveillance. Most importantly, many professionals (midwives included) convey private misgivings about screening in relation to its accuracy, its capacity to open a 'can of worms', and – for some professionals – its problematic relationship with 'eugenics' (namely on account of Down's syndrome being 'compatible with life'). However, much of their work involves silencing these values and interpretations, which links to how screening is downgraded in various ways: it is not prioritised since other tasks are privileged; it is not allocated time, money, and other resources; ultrasound scans are primarily cast as 'days out' rather than serious medical procedures, and so on. Whilst professionals express concerns about the practice on medical, socio-political, and moral grounds, screening for Down's syndrome persists, nonetheless, as a natural and routine part of a pregnancy.

In addition, despite professionals' anxieties and ambiguities about screening since Down's syndrome is 'compatible with life', everyday practices in the clinic render the condition absent in consultations. The symptoms, prognosis, and social realities of a future child with Down's syndrome are expelled from everyday routines. Since it is conventional to appeal for 'normal' children (Shakespeare 2011), the moral value of the foetus with Down's syndrome appears to have scant purchase in prenatal care. With the condition lacking a language of its own, it is colonised by universal negatives such as 'risk', 'problem', and 'abnormality'. This black-boxing masks the sizeable physiological and intellectual variation of people with the condition, acting as 'a stuff mould into which processes and beings must be made to fit even at the cost of distorting them' (Martin 1998: 126). The notion that people with Down's syndrome vary considerably is eclipsed, as well as the notion that disability more generally is shaped by cultural ideas of 'the normal' and a complex interplay of social, cultural, material, biological, economic, and political factors (Davis 1995; Ginsburg and Rapp 2013; Oliver 1990; Shakespeare 1999). Social conditions, indeed, can be as enabling or disabling as biological conditions. Taken together, such developments highlight the complexity of a practice in which Down's syndrome itself is constructed as 'compatible with life' in one moment and in another as a risk/problem (Chapter 5) and as a legally acceptable reason for termination (Chapter 6). For the most part, Down's syndrome is imbued with negativity and seems to hold a metonymical status as something which *can* and *should* be detected and, if a diagnosis is established, as something which constitutes a reason for terminating a pregnancy (Asch 1999; Burton-Jeangros et al. 2013; Rothschild 2005; Saxton 2013).

The prognosis for many genetic conditions, such as Down's syndrome, is frequently uncertain. A conclusive diagnosis rarely informs parents/parents-to-be about what their child will be like and, as such, much is left to their imagination when grappling with deep uncertainties that are likely to be shadowed by stereotypes of what it means to be disabled. Agreeing with Silverman (1987) that the illness of a child and ideas around both medicine and family/kinship are discursively constituted in consultations, I have shown how screening for Down's syndrome is downgraded and how the condition, before a diagnosis is established or suspected, is constituted as a negative, stigmatising, and innately problematic outcome. Here, there is an interesting twist on Lippman and Wilfond's (1992) 'twice-told tale'. Whilst Down's syndrome is described in the backstage of the clinic in positive terms, information provided in the frontstage of the clinic (in consultations) portrays the condition in more negative ways. It was claimed in Chapter 5 that the negative configuration of Down's syndrome in prenatal care may, in turn, represent *one* reason why termination rates in England and Wales have remained at around 92% for over twenty years.

The interesting and ironic paradox is that medicine, a discipline which can increase the life expectancy and quality of life of the child with Down's syndrome after he or she is born, also decreases the chance of a baby with the condition being born in the first place. The universal offer of Down's syndrome screening is a significant source of tension between medical/scientific communities and the disability community at large (Resta 2011). At this point, I emphasise that I do not subscribe to the argument that *all* population screening/testing equates to a negative valuation of disabled peoples' lives. This critique is predicated on the tension outlined above, namely that the medical/scientific community, by distinguishing 'normal' from abnormal', is perceived as placing the foundations for broader stigmatisations and discriminations against people with disabilities (Parens and Asch 2003). It is unhelpful and insulting both to professionals and parents-to-be who make difficult choices to use 'highly emotive rhetoric to denounce modern prenatal screening' (Shakespeare 1999: 682). This often manifests itself in claims that screening/testing is an egregious eugenic exercise evocative of Nazi Germany and that healthcare professionals responsible for delivering this programme are 'playing God' (Rock 1996: 121). This simplistic account disregards the complexity of an intricate issue, denies the meaning of impairment when conceptualising disability, and upholds unhelpful distinctions, such as 'eugenics vs. choice' (Duster 1990; Shakespeare 1999; 2000; 2011). It is tempting to identify prenatal screening as a tale of triumph or tragedy, of being wonderfully progressive or as nightmarishly evil. The reality, in truth, is much more complicated. As expressed in Chapter 5 particularly, screening for Down's syndrome is different than that for other conditions – such as Tay Sachs disease,[1] achondroplasia,[2] and Edward's syndrome – or screening parents-to-be with a family history of a genetic condition (Shakespeare 2000). It would be wrong, then, to indulge in exaggerated hype about *all* screening procedures translating to an 'old eugenics' (Kerr et al. 1998: 176).

But what about Down's syndrome screening? Analysing both the social and ethical issues ignited by genetic technologies, Duster (1990) explains that there are different drives for terminating a pregnancy and censures simplistic and unfair accusations aimed at the alleged eugenics of modern medicine. However, he also claims that whilst the 'front door' to eugenics appears closed, the 'back door' of disease and disability prevention remains ajar. Could it be that Down's syndrome screening keeps the back door ajar? I do not read screening, with Duster, as a planned plot against people with Down's syndrome and I do not entertain the argument that all terminations of pregnancy following a diagnosis are exclusively attributable to discrimination against people with the condition. Decisions are complex and can be made with reference to wanting to prevent suffering or a feeling that parents-to-be and their family will be unable to cope with the strain of caring for a disabled child (Korenromp et al. 2007). It may also be, of course, that parents-to-be undertake screening to 'prepare' for what they may perceive to be an unexpected and challenging situation, meaning that a diagnosis of Down's syndrome is not *always* viewed as 'unvalued' (at least by them).

However, the claims in this book suggest that a discussion about Down's syndrome screening through a lens of eugenics *can* be productive. Others have claimed that expanding options for reproductive selection – framed as a matter of individual choice and volition – constitute a refined version of twentieth-century eugenics (Lock 2007; Raz 2009; Taussig et al. 2003), with disability rights scholars critiquing prenatal techniques for reproducing implicit value judgements that disabled peoples' lives are worth less than other lives. Whilst I refrain from emotionally loaded accusations that *all* prenatal screening can be charged with promoting a eugenic agenda, I am equally wary of idealising prenatal care as an arena free of enacting particular morals and values around Down's syndrome. What I suggest is that, because we cannot consider screening and testing apart from its eugenic roots (Kerr and Cunningham-Burley 2000), it is fairer and more productive to assemble a division between 'historical eugenics', operating at the level of populations, and 'contemporary eugenics', operating at the level of individuals and families (Shakespeare 1995: 8–10). Shakespeare's (1998: 669) argument is that, whilst prenatal screening and testing do not translate to the old eugenics, the practices of reproductive medicine and the context under which reproductive decisions are made, particularly with respect to problematic cultural attitudes to disability, undermine the capacity for 'non-coercive individual choices' and can promote eugenic outcomes.

As shown in this book, Down's syndrome screening is arguably associated with the latter of Shakespeare's distinctions. In the context of the study, the race for a Down's syndrome diagnosis in the absence of a cure made possible by the availability of prenatal technology – and its routinisation in prenatal care – inadvertently serves as a commentary on which lives are valued and unvalued, and how particular ways of being in the world are threatened, stigmatised, and denied. Thus, the only option, particularly when there is no 'cure' or 'treatment' but only 'identification' and 'prevention' (otherwise known as the 'therapeutic gap'), appears to be to terminate the pregnancy (Alderson 2001; Asch 1999; Rothman 1998; Shakespeare 1999; Sooben 2010), with screening consultations becoming specific and salient outlets for the (re)production of Down's syndrome as a problematic and fearful outcome. According to McLaughlin (2003: 308), prenatal screening is part of a 'dangerous moral order' that constructs disability as 'removable and marginal, and the categories of the non-disabled as central'. This is not just about the morals of screening but concerns the politics of life itself (Rose 2006). At the 'entrance portals' of life, such techniques urge us to ask what kinds of people we will permit to be born or not and, by presenting Down's syndrome as a clear diagnosis, the message is that screening and testing is, essentially, for the purpose of termination (Rothman 1998: 117).

This is amplified by the routinisation of Down's syndrome screening and testing; 'the easier it is to blur the eugenic purpose of a technology, the more it is allowed to become routinised' (Ivry 2006: 460). The range of technologies available for detecting potentially disabling conditions has increased exponentially yet it seems that the fund of social knowledge accompanying such decision-making processes are limited (Ginsburg and Rapp 2013). Whilst such techniques can turn parents-to-be into moral gatekeepers, it seems that few people have an understanding about what it might be like to have, or live with someone who has, a specific disability (Franklin and Roberts 2006; Ginsburg and Rapp 2013) – including Down's syndrome. This emerges in conjunction with a spread of disability consciousness which offers support to families of children with disabilities (Finger 1999) and reports in both autobiographical and research literature that having a child with a disability, like Down's syndrome, is not the tragedy one initially expected it to be (Thomas

2015). Medicine, therefore, must take responsibility for ensuring that a fair and accurate depiction of conditions such as Down's syndrome is realised – rather than reinforcing any form of stigmatisation and/or discrimination.

It is unfair, however, to lay the blame entirely at the feet of professionals who face mounting pressures to 'meet targets and adhere to forms of clinical governance' that infiltrate the minutiae of clinical work (White et al. 2012: 79). Tensions between efficiency, economy, and care play out in everyday clinical life and whilst professionals – in an increasingly understaffed and under-resourced system – do play a role in the downgrading of Down's syndrome screening and how the condition is negatively constituted in prenatal care, they are not exclusively accountable for this. There are a number of heterogeneous elements which have combined to establish Down's syndrome screening as a routine affair and the condition itself as a negative life event, leading to accusations of constituting a 'contemporary eugenics'. This includes: a history of people with Down's syndrome being institutionalised and sterilised (and killed); the growth of clinical genetics and prenatal techniques; passing abortion laws; the failing policies of de-institutionalisation and community care; the medicalisation of pregnancy and the subsequent colonisation of reproductive care by clinicians; the acceptability of medical screening as a knowledge practice and our preoccupation with avoiding 'risks'; recommendations of prenatal self-care which understands foetal health as perfectible rather than as something largely determined through genetic and chromosomal constitution, and; current public discrimination and stigmatisation against people with disabilities (such as access to various resources). Many people, practices, and materials, then, are complicit 'in the reproduction of a given ideology' (White et al. 2012: 79).

Arguably, the technological path to identify and prevent the birth of a child with Down's syndrome, drawing on Ivry (2006: 459), is 'indexed as a backstage business because of a historically charged politics of disability'. This book captures how a negative depiction of the condition comes to life powerfully, and most effectively, in prenatal care. Although the conceptualisation of disability as a catastrophic outcome – that is, as 'the future no one wants' (Kafer 2013: 46) – is part of a broader discourse in the global North (Oliver 1990), it is particularly strong in the context of prenatal screening. This is undoubtedly driven by the medicalisation of pregnancy as part of the project of obstetrics that erects divisions between 'normal' and 'abnormal' pregnancies and future bodies (Hiddinga and Blume 1992; Olarte Sierra 2010). Obstetrics introduced the notion of 'potential abnormality' into practice by gaining knowledge of 'pathological' pregnancies that required treatment and diagnosis. Such categories of normal and abnormal remain today. As an indelible part of our medical and social culture, such technologies bring to life what counts as a 'normal' body.

This construction of the normal body is an extension of our society which seemingly privileges the mind over the body, identifying cognition as essential to personhood (Latimer 2013). The language of medicine claims to be neutral and universal yet it produces and reproduces rich, layered, and powerful messages via divisions of the normal and abnormal body (Rapp 1988; 2000; Vailly 2008); 'if you are not like everybody else, then you are abnormal, if you are abnormal, then you are sick' (Foucault 2004: 95). In Freymarsh and Springtown and in prenatal care more generally, Down's syndrome is similarly implicated in such 'dividing practices' (Foucault 1983) as abnormal, sick, and not like everybody else. The condition becomes embedded into a single class of 'abnormal' which shrouds the variable physical and intellectual difference of people with the condition under a blanket of universal and narrow categories. This, in effect, reduces its character and changes what people with Down's syndrome are or could become, thereby undercutting and problematising the choice purportedly promised by reproductive technologies:

> The choices promised by the advocates of the new human genetics are also highly circumscribed by the personal, clinical and wider social context in which they are offered. Bodies remain docile when the options for their reinvention follow the conventions of beauty and health; and reproduction remains a fateful process because of the very ability to eliminate the undesirable in favour of a norm.
>
> (Kerr and Cunningham-Burley 2000: 294)

Whilst Kerr and Cunningham-Burley concentrate on the new genetics, their claims are important here. This process of starting with routine care and ultimately facing questions about the meaning and value of human life, the life of one's potential child, is what Samerski (2015) calls 'the decision trap', that is, how engaging with genetic technologies can cause choices to become 'traps' that people enter both willingly and eagerly. Here, pressures surrounding the choice – the services available, expectations, cultural attitudes to disability, familial and other support, and so forth – interfere with this 'choice' being freely made. Lippman (1994: 19) argues that choosing to continue a pregnancy after a prenatal diagnosis of Down's syndrome 'cannot be considered a real option when society does not truly accept children with disabilities or provide assistance for their nurturance'. As such, rather than offering 'choice', we can suggest that Down's syndrome screening reflects a contemporary eugenics. The focus on identifying and preventing people with the condition, coupled with the development of reproductive technologies framed as bene-fitting the collective, bears much in common with the modernist project to efface and eradicate the Other; the desire for a 'perfect child' has become a common refrain, as has the alleged anguish and misery caused by genetic conditions (Kerr and Cunningham-Burley 2000: 291).

Prenatal screening intersects with social and cultural preoccupations with certain bodies, families, and desires (Latimer and Thomas 2015). Divisions of normal and abnormal, reproduced via the moral ordering work of contemporary hospital life, seem to enact the baby diagnosed with Down's syndrome as universally 'abnormal' and as unvalued by both medicine and the wider public (Ginsburg and Rapp 1995). By making Down's syndrome screening available, one can argue that this is already, by definition, problematising the birth of a child with the condition (Asch 1999; Alderson 2001; Lippman 1994; Rothman 2016) – and that such a life is interpreted as so onerous to the disabled child, family, and society that their avoidance becomes a public health priority (Wasserman and Asch 2006).

My focus on the ongoing negotiations of Down's syndrome screening in the clinic not only reveals the overt and covert inclinations toward selective reproduction but, also, challenges very simplistic or entirely beneficent readings of modern biomedical screening technologies. Prenatal screening and testing is a mixed blessing. It offers the possibility of detecting severe health conditions before birth and can prevent suffering for families, yet it can also induce great anxiety in parents-to-be and provide a running (moral) commentary on what lives we value. Reproductive technologies, thus, raise urgent and disquieting questions, for the public and professionals alike, about our ideas of 'normality', human variation, and when variation *becomes* a disability. This categorical work is vital to prenatal screening being continued. In order for screening to endure in its current form, Down's syndrome must be treated as abnormal and as an inherently negative outcome. One may argue, then, that parents may not necessarily be given an opportunity to take on the role of 'moral pioneers' as Rapp (2000: 3) describes in her seminal ethnography on amniocentesis. That is, the notion of 'choice' is problematic, if not entirely redundant, once Down's syndrome is constructed in such a manner. We can argue, thus, that Down's syndrome screening could be considered as a mode of contemporary eugenics, in that it effaces, devalues, and has the potential to prevent the births of people with the condition.

What next?

So what does the future hold for Down's syndrome screening? At the time of writing, non-invasive prenatal testing (NIPT) has just been introduced in the UK. This test is currently available in privately funded clinics and discussions are afoot to make NIPT the routine screening programme for Down's syndrome in the NHS. NIPT is used to analyse cell-free foetal DNA in a pregnant woman's blood at around ten weeks' gestation. It can accurately predict the chance of a foetus having a genetic condition like Down's, Edward's, or Patau syndrome; for example, at least 99% of all pregnancies in which a foetus has Down's syndrome can be detected using NIPT. Screening for sex chromosome disorders (for example, Turner syndrome) is also possible via NIPT. Although most pregnant women will receive a lower-chance (or 'lower-risk') result, some will have a higher-chance (or 'higher-risk') result, meaning it is highly likely that a foetus has a genetic condition. In such instances, diagnostic testing (CVS or amniocentesis) is used to validate this (i.e. NIPT is not officially classified as a diagnostic test). As NIPT is non-invasive, it presents no risk of miscarriage or other adverse outcomes associated with diagnostic tests.

However, many concerns about NIPT arise. For one, since NIPT is not universally available on the NHS, how will the service be delivered and is parity of provision a realistic goal, if a goal at all? How will NIPT be marketed by the companies selling it? How will this be regulated and what claims will be made? What impact will accessing privately funded clinics have for training healthcare professionals to deliver this programme? Since many studies on NIPT are funded by industry, does this invoke an implicit (or, perhaps, even explicit) bias? As this research has mostly been carried out among 'high-risk' populations, what happens once it is rolled out, as planned, in the NHS for 'low-risk' women? NIPT also intensifies long-debated issues in prenatal screening, such as assessing if 'non-directive care' and 'informed choice' are achieved and whether screening heightens anxiety. Yet other social and ethical questions may be asked of this new technology. For instance, since NIPT is reported as having a 99% detection rate for Down's syndrome, how will this knowledge be managed by pregnant women? Will this create added social and medical pressure to take tests – and does this affect a woman's ability to 'choose not to choose' (Kelly 2009)? What happens to 'choice' when screening is at an earlier gestation and 'risk' is diminished? Will women think less deeply about consenting to screening, thereby creating problems if they receive a result that they are not prepared for? How do pregnant women understand and handle inconclusive results as well as 'variants of uncertain significance' (variation in the normal sequence of a gene, the significance of which is unknown) and 'incidental findings' (undiagnosed medical conditions found unintentionally)?

It is also worth acknowledging that NIPT has the potential to detect genetic conditions other than Down's, Edward's, and Patau syndrome (Duchenne muscular dystrophy,[3] achondroplasia, thanatophoric dysplasia,[4] etc.). It may also be expanded to include next-generation sequencing[5] or microarray testing[6] that would make it feasible to screen for deletions and duplications in the foetal genome, including chromosomal imbalances too small to be detected via standard karyotyping (see: Chapter 2). In such a case, who decides what will be screened for? Will all identified genetic variants be shared with pregnant women? Do they have a right to access this information? How will they and professionals contend with the potential production of uncertain knowledge? Will NIPT be used 'inappropriately' (e.g. in cases of sex selection)? Will pregnant women receive support in the form of expert counselling to digest the results of testing for a large range of genetic diseases and disorders? How will the scientific community respond to these concerns among others raised by disability rights groups, like 'Don't Screen Us Out' and 'Saving Down Syndrome', vocally opposed to the development of new techniques of screening in fear that it extends an 'informal' eugenics? Since NIPT, in particular, has the potential to detect many different conditions and genetic variations, concerns about its eugenic potential – and the enduring negative valuation of disabled people – are particularly acute.

Such questions will only be answered in due course but do, indeed, require critical attention. An array of other scholars have reflected on the social and ethical issues associated with NIPT with more detail and nuance than is possible here (for an extended exploration of these issues and citations to this other work, see: Thomas and Rothman 2016). Whilst I make no grand claims about NIPT or what will come of it in this chapter, I reflect upon how the study reported in this book prompts crucial and challenging reflections on NIPT and the future (bio)politics of reproduction. For one, NIPT is likely to extend the dichotomy of normal/abnormal. In an era when human lives are increasingly measured and weighed in accordance with medical and scientific framings, notions of what is 'normal' have changed drastically – and the concept continues to haunt reproductive practices (Davis 2014). Indeed, there is a fear that 'the normal is shrinking' at the same time as our consciousness of the riskiness of reproduction is intensified (Latimer 2013: 192). As biomedicine extends its gaze, we are entering an era in which professionals must weed out certainty from uncertainty produced by modern prenatal techniques. With screening becoming more accurate, less invasive, and more widely available, the 'normal' is exposed by possibly detecting more genetic duplications, deletions, translocations, inversions, and insertions. As the body itself is more fully probed and finely enumerated, the category of the normal shrivels and the parallel category of the abnormal swells. It will be vital to track how medicine, built upon classification systems, handles this ambiguity in the context of NIPT and other developments that, in turn, lead us further down the path where we begin to consider who we will accept, or not, into families and wider society.

Similar to Down's syndrome screening at present – a practice which, as this book captures, has been entirely routinised in prenatal care – the controversies and complications of NIPT have also, mostly, been muffled. To illustrate this point further, we can draw a comparison with the public dialogues organised by the Human Fertilisation and Embryology Authority on mitochondrial transfer (HFEA 2013). The public dialogues were arranged to assemble views on emerging techniques, specifically on their social and ethical dimensions, designed to prevent parents from passing on genetically inherited mitochondrial diseases to their children. Cutting-edge reproductive technologies, Löwy (2014) argues, are often extensively debated by the media yet no such debates were, or have since been, organised regarding NIPT. The speed with which a technique spreads does not necessarily reveal its social acceptability, thus masking possible controversial social values embedded within it (Vassy 2005). The routinisation of Down's syndrome screening in many countries across the world, the UK included, has ensured that NIPT (like its predecessor) has not been subjected to public scrutiny, other than within the campaigns of the disability rights groups cited above. Indeed, despite some bold attempts, 'the debate has scarcely even started' (Clarke 1997: 128).

Instead, NIPT is viewed as an extension of an existing programme and an example of self-evident medical progress that smoothly follows the trajectory of earlier innovations: a mostly incremental and unexamined transformation of a new technique into a routine medical technology (Löwy 2014). Since Down's syndrome screening is so routinised, the diffusion of NIPT into clinical practice has been essentially untroubled and unchallenged, a subtle reconfiguration rather than a leap into a brave new world; 'where new tests fit old paradigms, uptake is higher and concerns are more mute' (Kerr and Cunningham-Burley 2000: 289). This reflects how the drive toward Down's syndrome screening 'appears to come from medical agencies, not from lay people or through democratic debate' (Alderson 2001: 362). With no UK parliamentary discussion on Down's syndrome screening, policies are formulated by advisory committees that emphasise preventing (alleged) suffering and promising informed choice. The risk is that NIPT, therefore, is viewed in the same way that Down's syndrome screening currently is: as a routine and mostly unproblematic procedure.

Although I have identified many concerns with screening for Down's syndrome throughout this book, I do not call for an end to reproductive choice or a ban on Down's syndrome screening. Indeed, my analysis has been about how screening is done and how it persists as opposed to whether it *should* persist. Prenatal techniques raise important questions around how technologies are used, regulated, and marketed, together with how they impact upon our conceptions of choice and responsibility and how both ethical and public concerns shape their development and diffusion. Yet our uncritical march toward scientific innovation renders the chance of putting a brake on the progress of Down's syndrome screening as incredibly slim. Once we know how to do something, it is difficult not to do it. Indeed, to quote a midwife cited earlier in the book (Chapter 5): 'once a screening test has been introduced, it's unlikely they'd take it away'. In the context of new methods of prenatal screening, we may be kindling a fire we cannot control. However, it is too late; the camel's nose is firmly in the tent since tests were 'developed, marketed widely, if not wildly, and changed our understandings of pregnancy, of foetal personhood as patienthood, in ways we cannot undo' (Rothman 2016: 1). Down's syndrome screening was introduced without serious public, scientific, and ethical debate, but we should think more about the new wave of biomedical innovations such as NIPT for Down's syndrome and other genetic conditions. This is particularly important in the knowledge that there were 687,852 births in England and Wales in 2015 (ONS 2016), highlighting the large number of mothers-to-be that would be offered the opportunity to undertake such practices in the future.

At this point, whilst I resist proposing specific policies to change and improve current practice,[7] suggestions worthy of deliberation – in conjunction with the questions outlined above – are proposed, thinking about NIPT particularly. As well as determining what or who is driving this practice, we should ensure that policies for NIPT and other forms of screening are reviewed through extensive, inclusive, and collaborative public debate that considers their consequences and implications before development and widespread diffusion. This should identify the need for the more careful and transparent regulation of prenatal techniques. In addition, pregnancy termination should be part of these conversations. For too long, termination has been divorced from debates about reproductive techniques. There is an explicit lack of public discussion of the (unspoken) practice of the 'selective' or 'therapeutic' abortion of pregnancy, yet it is intimately tied up with prenatal technologies such as NIPT. Already located in a context of secrecy and shame (Lotto 2015; Strange 2015), termination and its relationship with disability and medicine, whilst a difficult and problematic topic, needs to be at the forefront of debates around prenatal screening – rather than being solely about 'informed consent' and 'reproductive autonomy'. This will necessitate revisiting regulatory frameworks, too, such as our existing ambiguous abortion laws. Given that there is currently no legal restriction on what conditions may be screened for, nor how accurate this has to be, debates should consider whether legal frameworks need to be reconsidered in light of introducing NIPT into clinical practice.

What is more, debates should involve critical and fundamental discussions around the values embedded in the knowledge and practices of screening and testing. Rather than focusing exclusively on the reproductive autonomy, rooted in discourses of certainty and responsibility, that such techniques allegedly promise, we must genuinely engage with issues around Down's syndrome and what lives we value in modern healthcare systems and wider society. Skotko (2009: 823) fears that, as medical progress leaps ahead, people with Down's syndrome will slowly 'disappear' from society. We cannot say for sure whether this will happen but we can recognise how our ability to detect 'foetal abnormalities', and Down's syndrome specifically, may be more coercive than descriptive. It is vital to fully engage with concerns surrounding Down's syndrome and other disabilities as a 'fact of life' not always to be eliminated in the drive for a 'perfect baby' (Shakespeare 2011: 40). By lifting Down's syndrome specifically out of the medical context, this will make it possible to 'speak in other languages' about the condition so that parents-to-be can 'come to a decision from a more nuanced and knowledgeable position' (Rapp 1988: 155–156). Rather than focusing exclusively on abstract ideals such as autonomy and non-directive care when discussing how we can improve healthcare practices (Mol 2008), it may be better to explore how one conveys information around conditions such as Down's syndrome prior to screening (Bryant et al. 2001).

This connects with a need to develop a more nuanced and informed approach to prenatal screening and testing (Shakespeare 1999; 2011; Williams et al. 2005). We are entering an era in which we may eventually be able to screen and test, and potentially terminate, for not only 'serious' conditions but also for 'mild' conditions and late-onset disorders. As such, professionals must be allocated the time and provisions to be sufficiently trained so they can competently deliver NIPT with respect to knowing about the technology itself, the conditions screened for, and the limitations of medical knowledge (Shakespeare 2011), since NIPT will likely usher in more uncertainty. This will ensure that NIPT is not prematurely adopted in the NHS and will make it possible for parents-to-be to be given balanced (or 'as balanced as possible') information that is neither overly sentimental nor overly pessimistic (Estreich 2016) about conditions screened for in the UK.[8] This will provide them with a greater opportunity to successfully digest this data and make a decision which is right for them (Boardman 2010; Sooben 2010). As shown in this book, it is the implicit that is communicated in how screening is 'done'. The implicit mediates the information shared within medical work and installs both the need for a choice and *what choice* will be made. This means that we should invest money and energy not simply just into the science and technology of this practice but, also, into the training and support accompanying it that will help to offer balanced information and sufficient counselling (Shakespeare 2011), possibly with the involvement of disability charity organisations and other stakeholders. At this time, prenatal settings seem to provide little opportunity for people to discuss and explore their beliefs about disability (Bryant et al. 2006). This demands immediate attention if we want to move closer to promising truly 'informed' choice in a context where our conception of 'normality' diminishes and our conception of 'abnormality' expands (and we must be careful, of course, not to bundle *all* disabilities and 'diseases' together in debates around screening).

In order to ensure that this choice is, indeed, truly informed, we must also consider the wider social context in which screening is cultivated and diffused. In the UK, there has been an extensive implementation and expectation of disability cuts, with some estimating that disabled people risk losing over £28 billion in income support between 2013 and 2018 (PSE 2013) – and the human costs being even harder to calculate. In addition, there are recent reports of serious failings in NHS units dedicated to the treatment of people with disabilities, including the case of Connor Sparrowhawk (a.k.a. LB) who, in 2013, drowned in the bath of an NHS Assessment and Treatment Unit for adults with disabilities (to read more about this case, see: Hattenstone 2016). Following a report from Mazars, an audit firm, it was revealed that over four years, the NHS had failed to investigate the 'unexpected deaths' of 1,454 patients with learning disabilities or mental health problems, including more than 700 within a single trust. Such cuts and treatment of people with disabilities are undoubtedly fuelled by structural deficiencies and neoliberal ideals penalising the unproductive and dependent, whether on the state or others (e.g. family members). By possibly disrupting what it means to be a neoliberal subject – the discrete, reflexive, autonomous, and conscious individual capable of rational and ethical thought – the person with a disability can often be figured as in deficit and denied a personhood tightly wound up in ideas of economy and commodity (Skeggs 2011). Bodies are expressions of 'person-value' (Skeggs 2011) to the neoliberal world and as biomedicine is deeply implicated in neoliberal forms of rule, we can see who is or who is not valued. Such developments contribute, in turn, to the continuing negative valuation of people who are disabled. Thus, if we are to truly offer informed choice, there must be fundamental changes at a social structural level to ensure that people with disabilities are not subjected to stigmatisation and discrimination that excludes full participation in society, and that disability is recognised as a universal aspect of human life which does not constantly dominate the lives of people with a condition (Asch and Wasserman 2009; Ginsburg and Rapp 2013; Wasserman and Asch 2006).

With NIPT minimising physical risks and offering an earlier result, one suspects that the number of parents-to-be choosing to undertake Down's syndrome screening is set to expand, particularly given the plans to diffuse NIPT into NHS practice. As such, these concerns are a matter of urgency. Conversations about screening, even within some of the academic literature, revolve around the mainstream bioethical discourse of choice, freedom, and non-directive care – that is, ideological frameworks described elsewhere as fictions (Asch and Wasserman 2009; Bosk 1992; Rapp 2000). This discourse, focusing upon individuals rather than society more widely, legitimises public policy (Vassy et al. 2014) but glosses over the need for a critical engagement with many of the issues identified above that currently sit at the margins of public debate. Via detailed empirical insights into Down's syndrome screening and a continued dialogue between key stakeholders – including healthcare professionals, parents-to-be, policymakers, charities, academics, and people with personal experiences of Down's syndrome and other disabilities – we can reveal how NIPT is not a trivial, straightforward upgrade. Indeed, it needs extensive public deliberation that triggers new and unsettling questions (McLaughlin 2003) and that provokes and challenges, rather than simply relieves and mollifies, both policymakers and medical and scientific communities (Kerr and Cunningham-Burley 2000). This will address, if not ever completely eradicate, concerns over routinisation that emerge so prominently throughout this book.

Summary

By exploring how and why we are so invested in Down's syndrome screening, and what effects this has for those involved, the book illustrates how it is downgraded in everyday practices, thereby stabilising it as a 'routine' part of pregnancy, and how the condition itself is constituted as a negative life event. My intention, once more, is not to offer specific policies designed to change or improve practice. More modestly, I hope that my arguments will ignite more reflexive and pluralistic dialogues – and better communication between professionals, parents-to-be, and the wider public, as a result – around screening for Down's syndrome, along with other genetic conditions. We are aware that knowledge implanted as innovation, and absorbed by wider society, creates relationships, identities, and responsibilities. Screening and prenatal care, indeed, change the way that we think and act, and alter our perceptions 'of self and other, of normality and abnormality' (Lippman 1994: 9). Spilling beyond the biological and into public arenas and intimate lives, screening is a potent site for uncovering assumptions buried deep in medical work and for exploring how ideas around pregnancy, ethics, choice, diagnosis, care, disability, and parenthood play out in the everyday life of the clinic. In sum, by taking the politics of reproduction seriously, I reveal how analysing the 'terrible ordinariness' (Bosk 1992: xvii) of clinical life in Freymarsh and Springtown raises important questions for professionals, parents-to-be, governments, and sociologists alike. All ethnographies become social history and Down's syndrome screening will move on. However, many of the dilemmas identified here will remain the same – including how biomedical technologies are routinised and how they can serve as a commentary on what lives we value (or not) – and the cultural forms of the clinic will probably show remarkable stability (Atkinson 1995). With the development of increasingly sophisticated and accurate technologies showing no sign of abating, prenatal medicine will continue to transform and shape reproductive politics in the UK, and around the world, for the foreseeable future. We must remember that sociologists are valuable assets for making sense of such changes.

Notes

1 Tay Sachs disease is a rare and usually fatal autosomal recessive genetic disorder which causes progressive damage to the nervous system.
2 Achondroplasia is a common form of dwarfism.
3 Duchenne muscular dystrophy is a form of muscular dystrophy which gradually causes muscle degeneration and premature death. It mostly affects males, although females can be affected in rare cases.
4 Thanatophoric dysplasia is a severe and generally lethal skeletal disorder characterised by a disproportionally small ribcage, very short limbs, and folds of extra skin on the arms and legs.
5 Next-generation sequencing (NGS) is a catch-all term used to describe a range of different techniques that allow for DNA sequencing (defined as the process of separating the different pieces of DNA). The sequence reveals the kind of information that is carried in a particular DNA segment.
6 Chromosomal microarray analysis is a technique used to identify extra (duplicated) or missing (deleted) chromosomal segments (sometimes referred to as copy number variants). It can be used with living individuals who do not have a specific diagnosis (such as Down's syndrome) but who have unexplained developmental delay or intellectual disability, autism spectrum disorders, or multiple congenital anomalies.
7 Schwartz and Vellody (2016) outline strategies that professionals may adopt when communicating with parents-to-be about a prenatal risk assessment and/or a diagnosis of Down's syndrome.

8 In the US (Pennsylvania specifically), state legislature known as Chloe's Law dictates that the Department of Health provide updated, evidence-based information
on Down's syndrome – including support services, treatment options, and positive
outcomes – to parents-to-be who receive a prenatal diagnosis of the condition
(Caplan 2015). This law is said to challenge a governing ethic of value neutrality in
genetics by moving toward a more disability-friendly message. Interestingly, in
North Dakota and Indiana, legislation has been introduced to prevent a termination of pregnancy if it is sought *exclusively* because a foetus has been diagnosed with
Down's syndrome.

Bibliography

Alderson, P. 2001. Down's syndrome: cost, quality and value of life. *Social Science and Medicine* 53(5), pp. 627–638.

Asch, A. 1999. Prenatal diagnosis and selective abortion: a challenge to practice and policy. *American Journal of Public Health* 89(11), pp. 1649–1657.

Asch, A. and Wasserman, D. 2009. Informed consent and prenatal testing: the Kennedy-Brownback Act. *American Medical Association Journal of Ethics* 11(9), pp. 721–724.

Atkinson, P. 1995. *Medical Talk and Medical Work: The Liturgy of the Clinic*. Thousand Oaks, CA: Sage.

Boardman, F.K. 2010. *The Role of Experiential Knowledge in the Reproductive Decision Making of Families Genetically At Risk: The Case of Spinal Muscular Atrophy*. Unpublished Ph.D. Thesis, University of Warwick.

Bosk, C.L. 1992. *All God's Mistakes: Genetic Counseling in a Pediatric Hospital*. Chicago: University of Chicago Press.

Bryant, L.D., Green, J.M. and Hewison, J.D. 2006. Understanding of Down's syndrome: a Q methodological investigation. *Social Science and Medicine* 63(5), pp. 1188–1200.

Bryant, L.D., Murray, J., Green, J.M., Hewison, J.D., Sehmi, I. and Ellis, A. 2001. Descriptive information about Down syndrome: a content analysis of serum screening leaflets. *Prenatal Diagnosis* 21(12), pp. 1057–1063.

Burton-Jeangros, C., Cavalli, S., Gouilhers, S. and Hammer, R. 2013. Between toler-able uncertainty and unacceptable risks: how health professionals and pregnant women think about the probabilities generated by prenatal screening. *Health, Risk and Society* 15(2), pp. 144–161.

Caplan, A.L. 2015. Chloe's Law: a powerful legislative movement challenging a core ethical norm of genetic testing. *PLoS Biology* 13(8), pp. 1–4.

Clarke, A. 1997. Prenatal genetic screening: paradigms and perspectives. In: Harper, P.S. and Clarke, A. eds. *Genetics, Society and Clinical Practice*. Oxford: Bios Scientific Publishers, pp. 119–140.

Davis, L.J. 1995. *Enforcing Normalcy: Disability, Deafness, and the Body*. London: Verso.

Davis, L.J. 2014. *The End of Normal: Identity in a Biocultural Era*. Ann Arbor: University of Michigan Press.

Douglas, M. 1966. *Purity and Danger: An Analysis of the Concepts of Pollution and Taboo*. London: Routledge and Kegan Paul.

Duster, T. 1990. *Backdoor to Eugenics*. New York: Routledge.

Estreich, G. 2016. An open letter to medical students: Down syndrome, paradox, and medicine. *American Medical Association Journal of Ethics* 18(4), pp. 438–441.

Ettorre, E. 2002. *Reproductive Genetics, Gender and the Body*. London: Routledge.

Finger, A. 1999. *Past Due: A Story of Disability, Pregnancy and Birth*. Seattle, WA: Seal Press.

Foucault, M. 1983. The subject and power. In: Dreyfus, H.L. and Rabinow, P. eds. *Michael Foucault: Beyond Structuralism and Hermeneutics*. Chicago: University of Chicago Press, pp. 208–226.

Foucault, M. 2004. 'Je suis un artificier'. In: Droit, R.P. ed. *Michel Foucault: Entretiens*. Paris: Odile Jacob, pp. 90–135.

Franklin, S. and Roberts, C. 2006. *Born and Made: An Ethnography of Preimplantation Genetic Diagnosis*. Princeton, NJ: Princeton University Press.

Ginsburg, F.D. and Rapp, R. 1991. The politics of reproduction. *Annual Review of Anthropology* 20, pp. 311–343.

Ginsburg, F.D. and Rapp, R. 1995. Introduction: conceiving the new world order. In: Ginsburg, F.D. and Rapp, R. eds. *Conceiving the New World Order: The Global Politics of Reproduction*. Berkeley: University of California Press, pp. 1–18.

Ginsburg, F.D. and Rapp, R. 2013. Disability worlds. *Annual Review of Anthropology* 42(1), pp. 53–68.

Hattenstone, S. 2016. 'We never thought that he wouldn't come home': why did our son, Connor Sparrowhawk, die? *Guardian* [Online]. Available at: https://www.theguardian.com/society/2016/apr/02/never-thought-he-wouldnt-come-home-why-son-connor-sparrowhawk-die [Accessed: 7 August 2016].

HFEA. 2013. Mitochondria public consultation 2012 [Online]. Available at: www.hfea.gov.uk/9359.html [Accessed: 7 August 2016].

Hiddinga, A. and Blume, S.S. 1992. Technology, science, and obstetric practice: the origins and transformation of cephalometry. *Science, Technology and Human Values* 17(2), pp. 154–179.

Ivry, T. 2006. At the backstage of prenatal care: Japanese ob-gyns negotiating prenatal diagnosis. *Medical Anthropology Quarterly* 20(4), pp. 441–468.

Kafer, A. 2013. *Feminist, Queer, Crip*. Bloomington: Indiana University Press.

Kelly, S.E. 2009. Choosing not to choose: reproductive responses of parents of children with genetic conditions or impairments. *Sociology of Health and Illness* 31(1), pp. 81–97.

Kerr, A. and Cunningham-Burley, S. 2000. On ambivalence and risk: reflexive modernity and the new human genetics. *Sociology* 43(2), pp. 283–304.

Kerr, A., Cunningham-Burley, S. and Amos, A. 1998. Eugenics and the new genetics in Britain: examining contemporary professionals' accounts. *Science, Technology and Human Values* 23(2), 175–198.

Korenromp, M.J., Page-Christiaens, G.C., van den Bout, J., Mulder, E.J. and Visser, G.H. 2007. Maternal decision to terminate pregnancy in case of Down syndrome. *American Journal of Obstetrics and Gynaecology* 196(2), pp. 149.e1–149.e11.

Landsman, G. 1998. Reconstructing motherhood in the age of 'perfect' babies: mothers of infants and toddlers with disabilities. *Signs* 24(1), pp. 69–99.

Landsman, G. 2009. *Reconstructing Motherhood and Disability in the Age of 'Perfect' Babies: Lives of Mothers of Infants and Toddlers with Disabilities*. New York: Routledge.

Latimer, J.E. 2000. *The Conduct of Care: Understanding Nursing Practice*. Oxford: Blackwell Science.

Latimer, J.E. 2013. *The Gene, the Clinic and the Family: Diagnosing Dysmorphology, Reviving Medical Dominance*. London: Routledge.

Latimer, J.E. and Thomas, G.M. 2015. In/exclusion in the clinic: Down's syndrome, dysmorphology, and the ethics of everyday medical work. *Sociology* 49(5), pp. 937–954.

Lippman, A. 1994. The genetic construction of prenatal testing: choice, consent, or conformity for women? In: Rothenberg, K. and Thomson, E. eds. *Women and Prenatal Testing: Facing the Challenges of Genetic Technology*. Columbus: Ohio State University Press, pp. 9–34.

Lippman, A. and Wilfond, B.S. 1992. Twice-told tales: stories about genetic disorders. *American Journal of Human Genetics* 51(4), pp. 936–937.

Lock, M. 2007. Genomics, laissez-faire eugenics, and disability. In: Ingstad, B. and Whyte, S.R. eds. *Disability in Local and Global Worlds*. Berkeley: University of California Press, pp. 189–211.

Lotto, R. 2015. *Decision Making About Congenital Anomalies: How do Women and Their Partners Make the Decision to Continue or Terminate a Pregnancy Following Suspicion or Diagnosis of a Severe Congenital Anomaly?* Unpublished Ph.D. Thesis, University of Leicester.

Löwy, I. 2014. Prenatal diagnosis: the irresistible rise of the 'visible foetus'. *Studies in History of Philosophy of Biological and Biomedical Sciences* 47(Part B), pp. 290–299.

Martin, E. 1998. The fetus as intruder: mother's bodies and medical metaphors. In: Davis-Floyd, R.E. and Dumit, J. eds. *Cyborg Babies: From Techo-Sex to Techno-Tots*. New York: Routledge, pp. 125–142.

McLaughlin, J. 2003. Screening networks: shared agendas in feminist and disability movement challenges to antenatal screening and abortion. *Disability and Society* 18(3), pp. 297–310.

Mol, A.M. 2008. *The Logic of Care: Health and the Problem of Patient Choice*. New York: Routledge.

Olarte Sierra, M.F. 2010. *Achieving the Desirable Nation: Abortion and Antenatal Testing in Colombia (the Case of Amniocentesis)*. Unpublished Ph.D. Thesis, University of Amsterdam.

Oliver, M. 1990. *The Politics of Disablement*. Basingstoke: Macmillan.

ONS. 2016. *Statistical Bulletin: Births in England and Wales: 2015*. Newport: Office for National Statistics.

Parens, E. and Asch, A. 2000. *Prenatal Testing and Disability Rights*. Washington, DC: Georgetown University Press.

Parens, E. and Asch, A. 2003. Disability rights critique of prenatal genetic testing: reflections and recommendations. *Mental Retardation and Developmental Disabilities Research Reviews* 9(1), pp. 40–47.

PSE. 2013. '28 billion' benefit cuts for disabled people [Online]. Available at: www. poverty.ac.uk/disability-government-cuts-reports/%E2%80%98%C2%A328-billion %E2%80%99-benefit-cuts-disabled-people [Accessed: 7 August 2016].

Rapp, R. 1988. Chromosomes and communication: the discourse of genetic counseling. *Medical Anthropology Quarterly* 2(2), pp. 143–157.

Rapp, R. 2000. *Testing Women, Testing the Fetus: The Social Impact of Amniocentesis in America*. London: Routledge.

Raz, A. 2009. Eugenic utopias/dystopias, reprogenetics, and community genetics. *Sociology of Health and Illness* 31(4), pp. 602–616.

Resta, R. 2011. Are genetic counsellors misunderstood? Thoughts on 'The relationship between the genetic counselling profession and the disability community: a commentary'. *American Journal of Medical Genetics Part A* 155(8), pp. 1786–1787.

Rock, P.J. 1996. Eugenics and euthanasia: a cause for concern for disabled people, particularly disabled women. *Disability and Society* 11(1), pp. 121–128.

Rose, N. 2006. *The Politics of Life Itself: Biomedicine, Power, and Subjectivity in the Twenty-First Century*. Princeton, NJ: Princeton University Press.

Rothman, B.K. 1986. *The Tentative Pregnancy: Amniocentesis and the Sexual Politics of Motherhood*. London: Pandora.

Rothman, B.K. 1998. *Genetic Maps and Human Imaginations: The Limits of Science in Understanding Who We Are*. New York: Norton.

Rothman, B.K. 2016. Yes. Yes but. *Journal of Medical Ethics* [Online first].

Rothschild, J. 2005. *The Dream of the Perfect Child*. Bloomington: Indiana University Press.

Samerski, S. 2015. *The Decision Trap: Genetic Education and Its Consequences*. Exeter: Imprint Academic.

Saxton, M. 2013. Disability rights and selective abortion. In: Davis, L.J. ed. *The Disability Studies Reader*. 3rd edn. London: Routledge, pp. 120–132.

Schwartz, E. and Vellody, K. 2016. Prenatal risk assessment and diagnosis of Down syndrome: strategies for communicating well with patients. *American Medical Association Journal of Ethics* 18(4), pp. 359–364.

Shakespeare, T.W. 1995. Disabled people and the new genetics. *Genethics News* 5, pp. 8–11.

Shakespeare, T.W. 1998. Choices and rights: eugenics, genetics and disability equality. *Disability and Society* 13(5), pp. 665–681.

Shakespeare, T.W. 1999. 'Losing the plot'? Medical and activist discourses of contemporary genetics and disability. *Sociology of Health and Illness* 21(5), pp. 669–688.

Shakespeare, T.W. 2000. Arguing about genetics and disability. *Interaction* 13(3), pp. 11–14.

Shakespeare, T.W. 2011. Choices, reasons and feelings: prenatal diagnosis as disability dilemma. *European Journal of Disability Research* 5(1), pp. 37–43.

Silverman, D. 1987. *Communication and Medical Practice: Social Relations in the Clinic*. London: Sage.

Skeggs, B. 2011. Imagining personhood differently: person value and autonomist working-class value practices. *The Sociological Review* 59(3), pp. 496–513.

Skotko, B.G. 2009. With new prenatal testing, will babies with Down syndrome slowly disappear? *Archives of Disease in Childhood* 94(11), pp. 823–826.

Sooben, R.D. 2010. Antenatal testing and the subsequent birth of a child with Down syndrome: a phenomenological study of parents' experiences. *Journal of Intellectual Disabilities* 14(2), pp. 79–94.

Strange, H. 2015. *Non-invasive Prenatal Diagnosis: The Emergence and Translation of a New Prenatal Testing Technology*. Unpublished Ph.D. Thesis, Cardiff University.

Strong, P. 1979. *The Ceremonial Order of the Clinic: Parents, Doctors and Medical Bureaucracies*. Henley-on-Thames: Routledge and Kegan Paul.

Taussig, K.S., Rapp, R. and Heath, D. 2003. Flexible eugenics: technologies of self in the age of genetics. In: Goodman, G.H., Heath, D. and Lindee, M.S. eds. *Genetic Nature/Culture: Anthropology and Science Beyond the Two-Culture Divide*. Berkeley: University of California Press, pp. 58–76.

Thomas, G.M. 2015. Un/inhabitable worlds: the curious case of Down's syndrome. *Somatosphere*. Weblog [Online]. 29 August. Available at: http://somatosphere.net/2015/07/uninhabitable-worlds-the-curious-case-of-downs-syndrome.html [Accessed: 7 August 2016].

Thomas, G.M. and Rothman, B.K. 2016. Keeping the backdoor to eugenics ajar? Disability and the future of prenatal screening. *American Medical Association Journal of Ethics* 18(4), pp. 406–415.

Vailly, J. 2008. The expansion of abnormality and the biomedical norm: neonatal screening, prenatal diagnosis and cystic fibrosis in France. *Social Science and Medicine* 66(12), pp. 2532–2543.

Vailly, J. 2014. Genetic testing, birth, and the quest for health. *Science, Technology, and Human Values* 39(3), pp. 374–396.

Vassy, C. 2005. How prenatal diagnosis became acceptable in France. *Trends in Biotechnology* 23(5), pp. 246–249.

Vassy, C., Rosman, S., and Rousseau, B. 2014. From policy making to service use: Down's syndrome antenatal screening in England, France and the Netherlands. *Social Science and Medicine* 106, pp. 67–74.

Wasserman, D. and Asch, A. 2006. The uncertain rationale for prenatal disability screening. *American Medical Association Journal of Ethics* 8(1), pp. 53–56.

White, P., Hillman, A. and Latimer, J.E. 2012. Ordering, enrolling, and dismissing: moments of access across hospital spaces. *Space and Culture* 15(1), pp. 68–87.

Williams, C., Sandall, J., Lewando-Hundt, G., Heyman, B., Spencer, K. and Grellier, R. 2005. Women as moral pioneers? Experiences of first trimester antenatal screening. *Social Science and Medicine* 61(9), pp. 1983–1992.

Index

4D baby bonding scans 148, 166
5D photo products 148

'abnormality' 8, 107, 128, 130, 131,
    132, 134, 135, 143, 144, 145, 163,
    174, 176, 180, 181, 182
Abortion Act 1967 30, 33, 144, 168n9
abortion *see* termination
absence 88, 107, 114–8, 123, 127,
    130–1, 133–4, 166, 174
'accounting' practices of professionals 8,
    9, 77, 173
accuracy of Down's syndrome screening
    80–1, 108
achondroplasia 178, 183, 189n2
actor-network theory 9
'Aktion T4' euthanasia programme 28
ambiguity 163; of professionals concerning
    Down's syndrome screening 77, 80–3,
    108–13, 173, 176
amniocentesis 29, 30, 32–3, 36, 40, 66,
    67, 81–2, 84, 85, 102n2, 114, 115–16,
    126, 183; consultants' role in 52, 58;
    and informed choice 79; material/spatial
    organisation 64; miscarriage risk 33,
    60, 102n1, 116, 128–9, 151–2, 155
anencephaly 42n10, 102n2, 145, 167n1
anomaly scans 43n26, 89, 90, 117

baby/foetus terminology 8, 15, 16n4,
    143, 154–60, 164, 166–7, 175
banal, the 6–7
Berg, Marc 10, 58, 63
biomedicalisation 128
'black box' 118, 176
Body Clock Testing 152–3
bonding 148, 168n4
Bosk, Charles L. 58, 68, 71, 101, 110, 189

'can of worms' 81–2, 101, 108, 129, 176
cardiac scans 13, 17n13, 52, 71, 92–3,
    149; *see also* heart defects
care, organisation of 121–3, 174
'chance' 130–1, 135
chromosomal abnormalities 29–30
chromosomes 37
'civil inattention' 121; *see also* Goffman,
    Erving
classifications 8–9, 48, 49, 52, 58, 65,
    72, 110, 131, 143, 158, 163
cleft board (cleft lip/palate) 12, 164–7
community care 31–2, 180
'compatible with life' 1, 15, 16n1, 80,
    107, 108–13, 160–1, 162, 174, 176,
    177
constituting of classes 58, 72
consultants: role in diagnostic testing 51,
    52, 58, 100; role in Down's syndrome
    screening 48, 51, 52, 58, 71, 173,
    176
'cost-benefit' analysis of Down's
    syndrome screening 112–13
'couch', the 52–3, 61–2
Cunningham-Burley, Sarah 109, 181
curtains 63–5
CVS (chorionic villus sampling) 32,
    33–4, 36, 40, 126, 183; consultants'
    role in 52, 58; material/spatial
    organisation 64

dating ultrasound scans 49, 73n1, 89,
    90; *see also* ultrasound scans
defensive practice 122; *see also* litigation,
    threat of
deinstitutionalisation 31–2, 180
diagnostic testing 34, 39, 40, 82, 126,
    155–6, 182–3; consultants' role in 51,

52, 58, 100; development of 32–4;
FMD (Freymarsh foetal medicine
department) 12, 51, 128–9
'dirty work' 71
disability 180; discrimination 131, 177,
187; historical accounts of 42n1;
negative conception of 15, 109,
134–5, 175, 188; terminology 17n9;
welfare cuts 187
'disability public' 134
disability rights movement 131, 178,
183, 185
disability studies 112, 145
disciplinary power 8, 129; see also
Foucault, Michel
discourse 8–9
disposal 9–10, 14, 58, 77, 86, 88, 101,
160–7
doors 64–5
Douglas, Mary 58, 66, 151, 163
Down, John Langdon 1, 26, 27, 28
Down's syndrome 1; absence in prenatal
consultations 107, 114–27, 174, 176;
common symptoms 38, 126; the
condition 37–9; 'disappearance' of
people with 186; emotional reactions
of parents-to-be to diagnosis 149–50;
'face' 38, 119, 120, 149, 150, 166,
167; familiarity of 118–21; life
expectancy 39, 119, 125, 177;
negative discourses 15, 107–13,
119–20, 127–35, 143, 144, 162, 174,
177; occurrence rates 37; positive
discourses 112, 113, 114, 126, 133–4,
135, 160–1; professionals' knowledge
of 123–7, 174; prognosis 38–9, 126,
177; quality of life 16n1, 38, 110,
161, 174, 177; severity 127; socio-
history 14, 25–42; stereotypes 120,
177; stigmatisation of 112, 113, 133;
variability 131–2, 177; see also idiocy;
mongolism
Down's syndrome screening 1; accuracy
of 80–1, 108; consultants' role in 48,
51, 52, 58, 71, 173, 176; cost-benefit
analysis of 112–13; development of
34–6; downgrading of 14, 48, 49, 56,
57, 58–67, 71–2, 77–8, 88, 100,
121, 125, 174, 176, 177; emotional
response of parents-to-be to 2–3, 3–4,
68, 69–70, 81, 99–100; as a eugenic
practice 77, 80, 107, 108–13, 176,

178–9, 180, 183–4; future of 182–8;
low priority of 53–4, 61–2, 65, 71;
organisation of care 121–3, 174;
practices of 49–72; previous research
2–5; professionals' 'accounts' of 9;
professionals' ambiguity concerning
77, 80–3, 108–13, 173, 176;
routinisation of 48, 58–63, 72, 77–8,
101–2, 110, 111, 122–3, 132, 173–4,
179, 184; study outline 10–11;
training practices 56–7; uptake
rates 1–2
downgrading of Down's syndrome
screening 14, 48, 49, 56, 57, 58–67,
71–2, 77–8, 88, 100, 121, 125, 174,
176, 177
'dramaturgy' 7; see also Goffman, Erving

Edward's syndrome (Trisomy 18) 1,
16n2, 17n7, 37, 39, 40, 95, 102n2,
109, 110–11, 114, 115, 116, 117,
118, 120, 135n3, 156, 178, 182, 183
'elderly primagravidas' see maternal age
emotional nature of screening work
69–70, 72
empathy 70–1
et cetera principle 115; see also Garfinkel,
Harold
ethnomethodology 6; see also Garfinkel,
Harold
eugenics 27–8, 29, 30, 178; and Down's
syndrome screening 77, 80, 107,
108–13, 176, 178–9, 180, 183–4

'face', Down's syndrome 38, 119, 120,
149, 150, 166, 167
FAD (Freymarsh antenatal department)
11–12; absence of Down's syndrome
during consultations 114–23, 127;
checklist 121–3, 130; emotional
nature of work 70; informed choice
78–9, 83–6; material/spatial
arrangements 61–3, 65, 153; MCAs'
(maternity care assistants) roles 49;
midwives' roles 49–50, 51, 52–5, 58,
61, 71, 72; organisation of care
121–3; practice of screening 49–50,
51, 52–5, 56–7, 58–60, 61–3, 65–7,
68–71, 72; professionals' knowledge
of Down's syndrome 124–6, 126–7;
quadruple screening 80–1; risk
discourses 128–30; timeslots 71;

training practices 56–7; *see also*
    Freymarsh
family 50; at ultrasound scans 89, 90,
    94–5, 96
feticide 158–9, 160, 161, 168n12
FMD (Freymarsh foetal medicine
    department) 12; baby/foetus
    terminology 156–7; cardiac scans
    92–3; cleft board 164–7; diagnostic
    testing 51; disposal 163–4;
    emotional nature of work 69–70;
    material/spatial organisation 63–4;
    professionals' knowledge of Down's
    syndrome 124
foetal death 156, 157; *see also* feticide;
    miscarriages
foetal sex 29, 30, 89, 90, 94, 96
foetus/baby terminology 8, 15, 16n4,
    143, 154–60, 164, 166–7, 175
Foucault, Michel 8, 9, 87, 117, 129,
    153, 167, 181
Freymarsh 10; definition of 'at-risk'
    39–40; downgrading of screening 48;
    language barriers 87–9; material and
    spatial organisation 9; object of
    diagnostic testing 40–1; object of
    screening 39–40; power 8; quadruple
    screening 39; risk factors 39; *see also*
    FAD (Freymarsh antenatal
    department), FMD (Freymarsh foetal
    medicine department

Garfinkel, Harold 6–9, 77, 115,
    121, 126
gender attributes 96, 102, 174
genetic counselling 68, 109, 174
Goffman, Erving 7–9, 27, 31, 62, 80,
    83, 89, 97, 121, 126, 150

'hands-off work' 48
heart defects 38, 43n26, 64, 111–12,
    117, 124, 159, 164–5; *see also*
    cardiac scans
hereditariness 28, 127
heteronormativity 96, 102
higher-risk results 40, 81–2; FAD 51,
    56–7, 60, 63, 84, 115, 116–18,
    125–6, 155; incidence of 40; SAD 51,
    125, 126
humour: as coping strategy 70; and
    ultrasound scans 94, 98, 114–15
hybrid practice, ultrasound as 91

identity, professional 7–8, 67–71
'idiocy' 25, 30, 42n2; *see also* Down's
    syndrome
'immutable mobile' 122; *see also*
    Latour, Bruno
informality, and ultrasound scans 94,
    98, 102
informed choice 4, 14, 77, 78–80, 101,
    109–10, 161, 162, 173, 186;
    everyday practice 83–7; and
    language barriers 87–9; *see also*
    non-directive care
institutionalisation 26–8, 31, 180

Kerr, Anne 109, 181
kinship, reproduction of 89, 91, 96–8,
    101–2

language barriers 119; and informed
    choice 87–9
Latimer, Joanna E. 9–10, 58, 72, 88,
    118, 134–5, 181, 184
Latour, Bruno 9, 118, 122
learning disabilities 38, 125, 126, 127;
    NHS treatment failures 187
Lejeune, Jérôme 29–30, 42
life expectancy 39, 119, 125, 177
Lippman, Abby 174, 177, 181, 189
litigation, threat of 33, 122
lower-risk results 40; FAD 51, 60, 63,
    84, 115; SAD 51, 55
Löwy, Ilana 33, 42, 184

Markens, Susan 108–9
material/spatial organisation 173; FAD
    61–3; FMD 63–4; and power 9; SAD
    147–8
maternal age 2, 26, 29, 33, 41, 100,
    174; and expectations of perfection
    143, 150–4, 167
'matter out of place' 58, 176; *see also*
    Douglas, Mary
McLaughlin, Janice 144, 179
midwives: 'hands-on' work 65–7;
    ambiguity about screening 77,
    80–3; professional identity 67–71;
    roles in screening 49–50, 51, 52–5,
    58, 61, 71, 173, 176; training
    practices 56–7
miscarriages 53, 57, 71, 159; detection
    of high-risk pregnancies 35; following
    Down's syndrome diagnosis 2; risk of

screening procedures 2, 33, 35, 40, 60, 102n1, 116, 128–9, 151–2, 155
'mongolism' 25–31, 42n2; see also Down's syndrome
'mopping up' 68; see also Bosk, Charles L.
'moral pioneers' 81, 182; see also Rapp, Rayna
motility 9, 72, 88, 135, 176

Nazi Germany, eugenics programmes 28, 178
negative discourses about Down's syndrome 15, 107–13, 119–20, 127–35, 131, 133, 134, 143, 144, 162, 174, 177
neoliberalism 187–8
NIPT (non-invasive prenatal testing) 15, 182–6, 187, 188
non-directive care 4, 14, 77, 78–80, 83, 86, 87, 101, 117, 161, 162, 173; see also informed choice
normality 8, 59–60, 143, 144, 145, 163, 174–5, 180; see also perfection
NT (nuchal translucency) scans 17n12, 36, 89, 114; and informed choice 79, 86; SAD (Springtown antenatal department) 13, 50, 51–2, 55, 57, 71, 73n9, 144–5, 146–7, 150–1
nuchal translucency 43n26; see also NT (nuchal translucency) scans

obstetrics 50–1, 180

parents of children with Down's syndrome, positive discourses of 133–4, 136n4, 179
parents-to-be 16n3; emotional response to diagnosis of Down's syndrome 149–50; emotional response to screening 2–3, 3–4, 68, 69–70, 81, 99–100; expectations of perfection 143, 144–54, 167; information provision to 79–80; knowledge of Down's syndrome 123–4
Patau syndrome (Trisomy 13) 1, 16n2, 17n7, 37, 39, 40, 95, 102n2, 109, 110–11, 114, 115, 116, 117, 118, 120, 156, 182, 183
patient abandonment 101; see also Bosk, Charles L.
Penrose, Lionel S. 29, 30, 33, 42

perfection 109, 143, 144–54, 167, 186; see also normality
personality traits, and ultrasound scans 95–6, 102, 174
personhood 157–8, 163, 175, 188
positive discourses about Down's syndrome 112, 113, 114, 126, 133–4, 135, 160–1
power: disciplinary 8, 129; material and spatial organisation 9; micro-physics of 8; see also Foucault, Michel
pregnancy, medicalisation of 50–1, 128, 180
prioritising of clinical tasks 53–4, 61–2
'problem' discourses about Down's syndrome 107, 131, 132, 134, 135, 174, 176
professionals: accounting practices 8, 9, 77, 173; ambiguity concerning Down's syndrome screening 77, 80–3, 108–13, 173, 176; detachment 10, 159–60, 175; as focus of study 10–11; identity-work 7–8, 67–71; knowledge of Down's syndrome 123–7, 174; see also consultants; midwives; sonographers
'public secret' 121

quadruple screen 35, 36, 39, 49, 67, 116; inaccuracy of 80–1, 150, 151
quality of life 16n1, 38, 110, 161, 174, 177

Rapp, Rayna 9, 33, 81, 145, 150, 158, 182
reproductive politics 1, 16, 41, 189
'risk' discourses about Down's syndrome 107, 128–9, 130, 131, 151, 174, 176, 180
routinisation of Down's syndrome screening 14, 48, 58–63, 72, 77–8, 101–2, 110, 111, 122–3, 132, 173–4, 179, 184

SAD (Springtown antenatal department) 13–14, 67; absence of Down's syndrome during consultations 114, 123, 127; administrative staff 51–2, 67; Body Clock Testing 152–3; commercial environment of 100; emotional nature of work 70;

informed choice 86; material/spatial arrangements 62, 65, 147–8; NT scans 39, 80, 81; older mothers 151; practice of screening 48–9, 50, 51–2, 55–6, 57, 65–6, 69, 70–1; pregnancy goods 147, 148, 166; professionals' knowledge of Down's syndrome 123–4, 126, 127; risk discourses 131; social dimensions of ultrasound scans 77–8, 89, 90, 91–102; sonographers' roles 50, 51–2, 55–6; timeslots 71; training practices 57; *see also* Springtown

Saxton, Marsha 112–3

Shakespeare, Tom W. 134, 179

sonographers: ambiguity about screening 77, 80, 81; emotional labour of 100; professional identity 69, 70–1; roles in screening 50, 51–2, 55–6, 71, 173, 176; and the social dimensions of ultrasound 77–8, 89–100, 101–2, 173–4; training practices 57

Sparrowhawk, Connor 187

Springtown 10; combined screening 39; definition of 'at-risk' 39–40; material and spatial organisation 9; object of diagnostic testing 40–1; object of screening 39–40; power 8; risk factors 39; *see also* SAD (Springtown antenatal department)

sterilisation, enforced 28, 31, 180

termination: following Down's syndrome diagnosis 2, 32, 85, 108, 110–11, 112, 120, 131, 144, 154–5, 156, 157, 158–9, 161–2, 163, 164, 166, 175, 177, 178, 179, 186; US law 190n8; public attitudes towards 42n7; *see also* Abortion Act 1967

Timmermans, Stefan 145

training practices for Down's syndrome screening 56–7

Trisomy 13 *see* Patau syndrome (Trisomy 13)

Trisomy 18 *see* Edward's syndrome (Trisomy 18)

Trisomy 21 *see* Down's syndrome

Turner syndrome 29, 40, 42n5, 99, 110, 182

'twice-told tales' 177; *see also* Lippman, Abby

UK: deinstitutionalisation 31–2; welfare cuts 187

ultrasound scans 13; as a 'day out' 91–6, 101–2, 174; development of 35; DVDs 148; social dimensions of 77–8, 89–102, 158, 173–4; *see also* dating ultrasound scans

USA: amniocentesis 32, 33; institutionalisation 26; terminations, following Down's syndrome diagnosis 2

Williams, Clare 81, 157

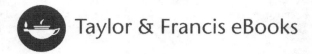

Taylor & Francis eBooks

Helping you to choose the right eBooks for your Library

Add Routledge titles to your library's digital collection today. Taylor and Francis ebooks contains over 50,000 titles in the Humanities, Social Sciences, Behavioural Sciences, Built Environment and Law.

Choose from a range of subject packages or create your own!

Benefits for you

» Free MARC records
» COUNTER-compliant usage statistics
» Flexible purchase and pricing options
» All titles DRM-free.

REQUEST YOUR FREE INSTITUTIONAL TRIAL TODAY

Free Trials Available
We offer free trials to qualifying academic, corporate and government customers.

Benefits for your user

» Off-site, anytime access via Athens or referring URL
» Print or copy pages or chapters
» Full content search
» Bookmark, highlight and annotate text
» Access to thousands of pages of quality research at the click of a button.

eCollections – Choose from over 30 subject eCollections, including:

Archaeology	Language Learning
Architecture	Law
Asian Studies	Literature
Business & Management	Media & Communication
Classical Studies	Middle East Studies
Construction	Music
Creative & Media Arts	Philosophy
Criminology & Criminal Justice	Planning
Economics	Politics
Education	Psychology & Mental Health
Energy	Religion
Engineering	Security
English Language & Linguistics	Social Work
Environment & Sustainability	Sociology
Geography	Sport
Health Studies	Theatre & Performance
History	Tourism, Hospitality & Events

For more information, pricing enquiries or to order a free trial, please contact your local sales team:
www.tandfebooks.com/page/sales

Routledge
Taylor & Francis Group

The home of
Routledge books

www.tandfebooks.com